DATE DUE

261-2500

Printed
in USA

THERE'S MORE TO BEING THIN THAN BEING THIN

NEVA COYLE

Authors of the bestseller *FREE TO BE THIN*

MARIE CHAPIAN

122748

BETHANY HOUSE PUBLISHERS

MINNEAPOLIS, MINNESOTA 55438

A Division of Bethany Fellowship, Inc.

Copyright © 1984
Neva Coyle and Marie Chapian
All Rights Reserved

Published by Bethany House Publishers
A Division of Bethany Fellowship, Inc.
6820 Auto Club Road, Minneapolis, MN 55438

Printed in the United States of America

Library of Congress Cataloging in Publication Data

Coyle, Neva, 1943-
    There's more to being thin than being thin.

    1. Reducing—Psychological aspects. 2. Reducing—Religious aspects. 3. Christian life—1960—
I. Chapian, Marie. II. Title.
RM222.2.C67 1984   613.2'5019   84-18587
ISBN 0-87123-443-2

The Authors

NEVA COYLE, Founder and President of Overeaters Victorious, makes her home in California with her husband and their three children. Educated in California and Minnesota, she attended Rasmussen School of Business and Lakewood Community College. She is presently working on her master's degree in Christian counseling. Neva has a busy speaking schedule across the country in seminars and media appearances.

MARIE CHAPIAN is well known as an author. Her long list of bestselling books include *Telling Yourself the Truth* and *Why Do I Do What I Don't Want to Do?* with Dr. William Backus, as well as *Love and Be Loved, Fun To Be Fit* and *Free To Be Thin.* Marie is a counselor and holds a Ph.D. in psychology. Her full schedule also includes radio and TV appearances and traveling and speaking throughout the USA and abroad.

Contents

Introduction

It's a blistering hot day in Redlands, California, and I am arriving at a meeting of people who have gathered to testify about the benefits of the *Free To Be Thin* program. I enter the church building where we are meeting, and find several women already inside. It has been four years since *Free To Be Thin*, the book about Neva Coyle's weight-loss program and her Overeaters Victorious plan, was published. Countless people have lost weight after reading the book and participating in the Overeaters Victorious (OV) weight-loss program. Thousands of letters have poured into the OV office as well as into mine, telling about lives changed, marriages strengthened and families united through the spiritual principles found in *Free To Be Thin*. These letters are a far greater measure of the book's success to Neva and me than merely the sales figures.

As I sit and wait for the meeting to begin, my longtime friend, Neva Coyle, approaches and sits beside me. She looks lovely and cool in her belted summer dress. (She once told me one of her greatest goals in life was someday to wear belts.) You would not call her skinny. Neva is what one would consider "average." I remember her telling me over five years ago, "Marie, all I ever wanted to be was *average*. I was so sick of wearing a raincoat to cover my fat even when it was hot. I was so tired of wearing size 24 overblouses every day of my life. My dream and my life's desire was to be *average*." Now I look at my "average" friend sitting next to me and I smile to myself.

"You look great, Neva," I tell her.

"Thank you," she responds, her smile an expression of her genuine warmth and joy. "I feel better now than I have ever felt in my life. In fact, things just keep getting better and better."

By now the people are assembled and I notice there is only one man in the group, certainly a thin one. Later I will learn he has lost 112 pounds on the *Free To Be Thin* program.

We make a circle with our chairs and begin the session. As the women respond to my questions, I realize each one probably represents countless other people with similar stories. Consider Belinda, for example. Belinda weighed 400 pounds when she discovered *Free To Be Thin*. In three years' time she has lost 81½ pounds. She still has many pounds to lose, but there is no frustration or guilt in her voice when she speaks about losing weight.

"Three years ago I didn't think anyone would ever love me," she begins quietly. "I thought I was just a misfit and always would be. I wasn't happy being myself and I wasn't happy trying to be someone else. I have been a Christian all my life, and I just never dreamed I could conquer my weight problem. I was only 29 years old and I was on my way to weighing a quarter of a ton!"

Tears form in Belinda's eyes, and the rest of the group listens and nods knowingly. Each of them knows the feelings of alienation, loneliness and despair that obesity can bring.

"Because I was overweight, I felt it was my duty to do

things like dieting."

I ask her how many weight-loss programs she has tried.

"How many are there?"

She had tried every weight-loss program imaginable without success. Now the tears drip down her cheeks. "When you come from a family who all weigh over 300 pounds and you believe you will always be fat and a misfit, you never have a feeling that when someone tells you they love you, they really mean it."

She then tells us how she was once the heaviest of her family until her younger brother passed her. He could not weigh himself on anything but a commercial scale because he was over 450 pounds. Belinda struggles to speak through her tears, "It's so wonderful because he lost 55 pounds in thirteen weeks through the *Free To Be Thin* program. I'm crying because I finally see hope, and I'm so—*so* grateful."

Jean from Riverside tells us how she lost 58 pounds in five-and-a-half months. Alberta joyfully explains she once weighed 202 pounds, and now her five-foot two-and-a-half-inch frame weighs 122 pounds. Mary tells of losing 48 pounds, and Barbara of 165 pounds.

You would think we are celebrating thinness, the beauty of slim bodies, but that is not what this book is about. Neva explains, "Losing weight is what we discover on the way to finding something else." She tells of looking for thinness and discovering something *more*. That is why we have called this book *There's More to Being Thin Than Being Thin*.

Is there really more than the freedom to be thin?

Belinda says she knew the answer to every question about losing weight. Why couldn't she change before now? Why was she so fat at 29 that she couldn't buy her clothes even in a "queen-size" store? She had read all of the diet books and tried all the programs. She could recite the number of calories in nearly any edible, but everyday life did not match her knowledge. There had to be *more* than thin. For her, knowing how to be thin was not enough and getting there was not enough either.

Once You're There

Many people *reach* goals, but skill, a special ability, is needed to *maintain* that goal. Lavonna, who has lost 25 pounds, says she once spent more time wishing she were tall so she could eat more than she did thinking about eating less as a short person. "My success depends on my commitment, and I really have always found commitment very difficult."

Lavonna tells us she never felt able to be the person God desired because she was overweight. She thought God would never use her because she felt so bad about herself. It was difficult for her to read *Free To Be Thin* and believe it was written just for her. Every time she had lost weight in the past, she had regained it. She had even taken a job with a weight-loss organization, thinking that would help her. It didn't. She only gained more weight and twice as much guilt.

Even if you have never read *Free To Be Thin*, or attended an Overeaters Victorious group, you will be helped by this book. When she began Overeaters Victorious, Neva wanted people to lose weight without having to join a weight-loss group. Thousands of people have lost weight in OV groups, but thousands have also lost weight just by reading and applying the principles of *Free To Be Thin* and the accompanying materials to their daily lives.

This book will encourage you and show you that you *can* lose weight and keep it off. Barbara's words, spoken slowly as she fought against tears, express what we are praying this book will do for you: "I have lost 165 pounds and I feel so much better about myself. I have changed, and *so has my whole life*. Being on the *Free To Be Thin* program is not something I do one day and don't do the next, because now I *am* free to be thin."

Barbara is still overweight, having more than 100 pounds to lose. "I still feel fat, but I am actually at a point in my life where I can think about things like being accepted and possibly one day getting married. Believe me, when I weighed nearly 400 pounds, marriage was not an option. I'm 32 years old and I've begun taking voice lessons and seeing that my life actually has a future!"

Even if you are not overweight, this book will help you. Not all the letters we receive are from overweight people. That is because we are aiming toward *more*, and that *more* is for you.

Marie Chapian

one

Free to Live

When Barbara weighed almost 400 pounds, she refused to enter a neighborhood store, afraid of being taunted by teenagers or children. Even now, after losing 165 pounds, she is hesitant to be around young people who might laugh and point and call her names. But she's stronger than ever.

"I know I am becoming the real me," she says. "In fact, I'm becoming *more* than the real me. I'm not thin yet, but I'm not afraid anymore. I'm not afraid to try new things—to live! I used to think I was born to watch TV and do needlepoint. Now I am shocked to discover I love to do things like go fishing. I even enjoy walking. I'm not ashamed to be myself."

Becoming the real you includes not only the things you enjoy doing, but also your feelings, thoughts and goals.

Another woman, Mary, tells how she had reached the point where she was ready to follow a group promoting being and staying fat. She says:

I was beginning to accept myself as I was because I didn't want to be depressed or frustrated. I was fat, and I looked and felt bad. It was not a good feeling to be left out and isolated, but that's what I was. I thought the solution was to accept myself as fat and undisciplined. I thought maybe

15

I could become less inhibited that way. Then I discovered
Free To Be Thin.

Carol, who lost 53 pounds, recalls trying to convince
herself fat was beautiful:

> . . . but who was I kidding? Fat is *not* beautiful. *Healthy*
> is beautiful. Even Gloria Steinem, the feminist leader, is
> not fat. I mean, if there would be one person who would
> advocate fat for the woman—to be free and herself, it's
> Gloria Steinem. But she battles overeating and stays thin.
> No, fat is not beautiful and nobody is free when he's fat.

Whenever I ask women, "Do you consider yourself bad
when you overeat?", they answer *yes.* Carol admits:

> Honey, I'm bad when I overeat, when I overspend, when
> I overtalk, when I overwork, when I oversleep, when I
> overdress. I simply cannot explain what it means to me
> to realize how many areas of my life I have hated.

June tells this tragic story:

> I have chosen to live alone, all by myself—that way no-
> body will be around me to show me all the flaws in my
> personality. Nobody will be around to remind me how
> unacceptable I am. I can keep people from getting close
> enough to me to discover all my problems. It never occurs
> to me that someone might like me and accept me as I am.

Slowly June is changing. She is now able to say, "I
have over 100 pounds yet to lose, but I consider that sec-
ondary. My every thought and hope is no longer in losing
weight. It's to see myself clearer as a lovable child of God."

Mold Me and Make Me . . .

When Neva Coyle asked the Lord to help her lose
weight, she also asked Him, "What *can* I eat?" God was
faithful and showed her what foods were good to eat. Then
one day she felt He was showing her it was not *what* she
could eat but *if.*

Have you ever heard anybody erroneously tell you the

way to know the Lord's will is to get everything you asked for? The truth is, if you are asking God a question and not getting an answer, it may have something to do with how you're allowing yourself to be molded by Him. In 1 Corinthians 10:13 the Apostle Paul writes:

> No temptation has overtaken you but such as is common to man; and God is faithful, who will not allow you to be tempted beyond what you are able, but with the temptation will provide the way of escape also, that you may be able to endure it.

It is difficult to know how to handle the blessings of abundance unless you are molded into the thought and mind of God. There is no temptation too big for you to handle. The Lord promises you that. Your situation is unique but God also tells you you're not alone. He is faithful and there to help you. He uses the perfect tools to pound, chisel and shape you to the "shape" with which you will be most happy. As you let Him work on you, you can dare ask Him questions like, "Lord, what should I eat?"

You probably tend to fix your attention on the temptations you are struggling with and becoming obsessed with them. If, at the onset of the temptation, you start looking for a way of escape, you will have to start with remembering what He has told you already. He has promised He will provide a way of escape—but what does this mean? For the overeater the escape route is very special.

One of the main escapes from eating the wrong food, and too much of it, is *knowledge*. Understand what you are doing. Neva tells victoriously of how she learned the truth about certain foods and was then able to eliminate them from her shopping list forever. Take Kool-Aid, for example: "My children have lived for three years without Kool-Aid in our house," she told the group. "I read that the sugar, artificial flavoring and colorings are bad for children who have a tendency to be hyperactive. That was all I needed to know. Out it went. My children have learned to drink orange juice and apple juice, and even water." Knowledge provided a way of escape.

"I'll never serve my family Jell-O again," one lady tells us. "I read the box and I was shocked at the amount of sugar in it. To think I always thought it was a diet food!"

Another woman says, "I don't eat luncheon meat anymore! The sodium nitrate and coloring is just not what I want in my body. I'm so glad I've learned to read wrappers!"

Another adds, "Yes! I've given up bacon because I read the wrapper—and diet soda, too!"

And another says, "And bags of chips. Was I shocked when I learned how much more than corn was in that bag. No more, let me tell you. From now on it's sliced apples for this Free To Be Thin person."

Becoming the real you requires gaining knowledge. You begin to see the real God as big enough to care about you and help you learn what's in the foods you eat. Did you know God can provide a way of escape when there is fattening and unhealthy food around every corner? He shows what is good for you and then makes sure it's available. At a luncheon there'll be salads just for you, hiding behind the no-no breads. There will be lean meats, vegetables, fruits, all healthy and waiting for you if you look for them.

The Holy Spirit guides and protects you. If you can agree with us that overeating has a spiritual solution, then you'll have to agree you can't solve it in your own strength or simply by your willpower. You might get thin by using willpower, but you won't gain a spiritual victory. You need a Spirit more powerful than your own to help: God's Holy Spirit.

One lady recalls her desperation:

I came to the end of my rope. I had nowhere to turn. I had gone without breakfasts and lunches, eating only small dinners, but I still gained weight. I tried liquid diets and tried total abstinence. Nothing worked. I didn't know how I could escape from the awful prison of my own overeating behavior. I can't even consider it appetite. I don't ever remember in all my years of hassling with overweight that I was ever really *hungry*.

The Holy Spirit is your escape because God has not only given you knowledge, He has given himself as an escape from your temptation. How big is God, you may ask? We answer, how big is your temptation? God is bigger.

Is Overweight a Spiritual Problem?

"I feel as though two poeople are fighting inside my body. One of me wants to have self-control; the other one wants to eat a dozen chocolate chip cookies." These are the words of a lady trying to lose weight using sheer will-power. It's admirable to have willpower, but we have found, as this lady is discovering, it is simply not enough. We need Holy Spirit power to attain what God intended us to be and have. Without Him, sooner or later we will give in to the cookies or the hollandaise sauce.

God says you can be a winner and overcome every sin and temptation. But you will never understand your true place in life until you see yourself with God's eyes. A. W. Tozer wrote, "The essence of idolatry is the entertainment of thoughts about God that are unworthy of Him." It is unworthy of God to exclude Him from any problem you might have. Any problem involving your unbridled appetites involves sin, and ". . . while we were yet sinners Christ died for us" (Rom. 5:8). God has the solution for every sin and problem you may face, including overeating.

There comes a point where you must believe God truly loves you and that He gave a Savior to take the punishment for every one of your bad behaviors. Will you believe Jesus gave His life for you so you can live in victory by the power of His Spirit? Will you yield yourself to His lordship and accept Him as Savior in every area of your life? You need spiritual power to overcome spiritual problems, and there is no problem you will ever encounter that God cannot help you overcome.

Pray: "Lord, I need help again. I am ready to repent, to turn from trying to overcome my problems with my own willpower. I realize I must have your supernatural power, so I ask you, Lord Jesus, to save me from myself. I return to you, my own personal Savior, and yield all of myself to you. I give you my body, soul and spirit to mold and shape. I believe I am your child because I have asked you to be my Lord. Fill me with your Holy Spirit anew and give me new life. Help me become the real me. In Jesus' name, amen."

two

Leaving the Past Behind

God's promises are true. He wants you to enjoy your life, to enjoy being you. He provides an escape from temptation, and as a Christian, you have personal access to that provision. As a Christian you can take God at His word even though it may seem impossible. You can dare to believe the truth. We believe that the answers to all our problems are spiritually based and found in God himself. He has promised a way of escape from temptation.

You are going to learn in this book how to focus your attention on the escape instead of the temptation to believe you are just a weak so-and-so who can't walk past a bakery or an ice-cream store without entering.

The Way You Were

And you were dead in your trespasses and sins, in which you formerly walked according to the course of this world, according to the prince of the power of the air, of the spirit that is now working in the sons of disobedience. Among them we too all formerly lived in the lusts of our flesh.—
Ephesians 2:1–3a

Notice the passage is past tense. You *were* dead, you *formerly* walked, you *formerly* lived. This is the way you

21

were *before* you gained understanding and gave your entire life to Jesus Christ. You tried to overcome problems but couldn't. You couldn't help but miss because you didn't use the power to succeed. Now you have an escape. You have the power of God within you, as well as an understanding of that power.

The Power of Mercy

But God, being rich in mercy, because of His great love with which He loved us, even when we were dead in our transgressions, made us alive together with Christ (by grace you have been saved), and raised us up with Him, and seated us with Him in the heavenly places, in Christ Jesus.—Ephesians 2:4–6

If you see the word *mercy* you probably think of kindness. You're right. The dictionary defines mercy as "compassion or forbearance shown to an offender." That's kind, isn't it?

When you accept God's mercy you can better accept yourself. Mercy can't be received by someone who won't admit he or she has done wrong. God has mercy on you, not because you are so terrific, but because He created you as an object of His love, and even though we have offended and wronged Him, we've found favor in His eyes because of Jesus' death on the cross.

Before you were a Christian person it was okay to use excuses like, "I'm just naturally fat. My mother was fat and my father was fat, so I'm fat." But now you cannot say something like that truthfully. Now you have a new parent; you have a heavenly Father. Bertha comments:

I have been a Christian all my life. My father was a minister and I have always gone to church and been involved in Christian activities. I just never knew that God could be concerned about my overweight. My mother and father are both overweight and my brother and sister are too. I always thought it was carnal to be concerned about my body, so I got fatter.

Bertha has learned now it is carnal *not* to be concerned about her body. She has learned God cares about her weight. She has learned it was far more carnal to be self-conscious and worried about the way she looked, that she was selfish when she fretted over being fat rather than give her weight problem to the Lord.

Jeanie, 39, who went from 212 pounds to 160 pounds, tells how she felt imprisoned as an overweight person:

> I'm five-eleven so I can carry more weight, but I have always felt embarrassed about being fat. My husband is younger than I, and that made me twice as self-conscious. I would sit in the back pew of the church so I could get out before everyone else. I didn't want anyone to see me. I felt fat. Fat and old.

Where does the Lord fit into all of this? Jeanie remembers eating a loaf of bread at a time and hating herself for it. "I think I have always been chubby. I lost weight for my wedding but it wasn't long before I was chubby again. It started at the wedding reception with the wedding cake."

Maybe you think you are one of those people who marches to a chubby drummer, but you have a Savior who is playing a new song for you. And whether you became a Christian five minutes ago or five decades ago, God cares.

Many Free To Be Thinners were raised in homes where fattening foods were a way of life. Almost every overweight person who has been through the OV program has had to learn a total new way of eating. Alberta, who lost 60 pounds, doesn't remember going to bed as a child without a snack (of up to five pieces of cinnamon toast). Bertha groans and confesses:

> I learned to believe I would die, or at least faint, if I didn't eat something every two hours. I was taught I needed to eat to keep my strength up. I guess I needed a lot of strength because at 16 I weighed 202 pounds and I'm only five foot two.

Putting the Past in the Past

What is the way you *were*? Were you that person sitting in the back pew at church? Were you the one who worked in the back room at your office? Were you in the back row of your choir hiding behind the tenors? Were you the one alone in the front seat of the car? Or home watching TV year after year, instead of meeting new people and going places? Is this the way you *were*?

We are talking about the past. Ephesians 2:1 says you *were* dead in your trespasses and sins. Now you *are* alive in victory because God, who is rich in mercy, loves you. You have been raised up to sit with Him in heavenly places with Christ Jesus. Repeat these sentences:

1. Failure is *past* tense for me.
2. I *was* helpless to overcome overeating, but not anymore.
3. I have found the way of escape through Christ Jesus.

You were once a slave of your old, former nature which was prone to sin and failure. Now, by working hand-in-hand with God toward a happier and more fulfilled life, you can become all you were meant to be. The Lord says you were created "for good works which God prepared beforehand that you should walk in" (Eph. 2:10). At one time you may have been a stranger to God's promises without hope. Now, however, you're no longer "far off," but "brought near" by the blood of Christ (Eph. 2:13).

Can you see the dramatic contrast between your old self and your new self? Now you can control those things of the past that hurt you. Now you can enter God's beautiful plan for your ultimate best. Your body will consistently reduce to the beautiful state that God has intended for it, because you will no longer be deceived by rationalizing and lying to yourself.

> **When you look for satisfaction in your life,**
> **you probably won't find it.**
> **When you seek God,**
> **you will find satisfaction.**

How many times have you resisted a meal and thought you'd starve to death? How many times have you awakened in the night and prowled hungrily into the kitchen for something to eat in order to satisfy your appetite? Satisfaction is always illusive when you hungrily pursue and feed it.

We make it very plain in OV that *you* are responsible for your own behavior. Most people seek satisfaction outside themselves. They say to food, "*You* make me happy." They say to friends and loved ones, "*You* give me what I need." They say to their work, "*You* give me a sense of fulfillment and satisfaction." They say to God, "How come I'm not satisfied? Did *you* make a mistake with me?"

The compulsive spender pursues satisfaction in buying things; the overeater looks for satisfaction or comfort in eating or being full. The spender surrounds herself with things; the eater fills herself with things. They are both materialists. Luke 12:29–31 gives an antidote:

> *And do not seek what you shall eat, and what you shall drink, and do not keep worrying. For all these things the nations of the world eagerly seek; but your Father knows that you need these things. But seek for His kingdom, and these things shall be added to you.*

You will have satisfaction in your life when you believe God to provide all you need. Only He can provide lasting satisfaction. Do the following:

1. Tell God you want to find your satisfaction in Him.
2. Tell yourself you are going to be responsible for your behavior.

If this seems simplistic to you, stop and recall how often you have blamed your overeating on somebody or something else. God may not remove the temptation to overeat, but He will provide the strength to meet it. In order to face temptation, you must admit that you, and you alone, are responsible for your response to temptation.

Suppose you have just finished eating at a restaurant and are still hungry, feeling unhappy and unsatisfied. Suddenly you think, *Did God really say I couldn't eat chocolate cake?* Your friends are eating dessert and so are the people at the next table. You spot two thin people eating enormous sundaes in a booth behind you. Again you think, *Where does it say in the Bible that chocolate cake is a sin?* That does it.

After you have polished off the chocolate cake and tasted the dessert of everybody else at the table, your mind swims with thoughts of other desserts. You can hardly wait to see if there is any ice cream in the freezer at home. Once there, you eat the ice cream, then attack the jar of jam in the refrigerator and eat every drop of it, as well as 13 cookies. "Why, oh why," you ask miserably as you fall into bed, "did my friend ask me if I wanted dessert? Wasn't it obvious I'm trying to lose weight?" That is shifting the blame on someone else.

You're more than thin when you can face temptation realistically. The Living Bible says, "But remember this— the wrong desires that come into your life aren't anything new and different. Many others have faced exactly the same problems before you. And no temptation is irresistible. You can trust God to keep the temptation from becoming so strong that you can't stand up against it" (1 Cor. 10:13).

You may think that if you have once given in to temptation, the above words will no longer apply to you. You may shrug your shoulders and say, "Oh, sure, that's great for valiant Christians who are much stronger than I," but your temptation to overeat is not unique. You are not alone.

You and Temptation

Recall the last time you were tempted to eat something you shouldn't have. What is the first thing that happened? Before you reached for that food you knew would not bless your body, you had to *imagine eating it*. It's difficult to understand this subconscious event because these thoughts may be only in images. Tests have shown that an over-weight person responds physically to the mere mention of food. (The average-weight person's response is much more moderate.) One group of overweight men and women, accustomed to overeating, would salivate at the smell of food cooking. When questioned, their response was a vague, "I thought the smell was pleasant," but most of them could not identify specific thoughts, such as, "I must eat that." It's important to train yourself to stop thinking how delicious and wonderful foods are, when certain foods are not so wonderful at all.

If you are asking God to help you lose weight or maintain your new, lower weight, He will answer that prayer because He is completely faithful. First Corinthians 10:13 says, "God is faithful." Your first temptation isn't really food; it's doubting that God can do what He says He will. Eve's temptation in the Garden of Eden really had very little to do with the fruit. Her temptation was to disbelieve what God had said. Satan said to her, "Did God *really* say you couldn't eat of that tree?", tempting her to doubt God.

> **It was lack of faith
> that caused the fall of man,
> not an apple.**

You may say to yourself, "God won't love me any less if I'm fat," as you head for the refrigerator, but this violates the prayer of faith you prayed when you asked the Lord to help you lose weight. He is faithful and He will always do His part when you allow Him to.

Before you can resist temptation again, tell yourself, "Yes, God is faithful." Now, look in your refrigerator and see what will tempt you. If it is full of foods that hurt rather than bless your body, can you trust the Lord enough to help you remove them? Can you trust the Lord to show you the foods to eat that are going to bless you?

Is God Angry with You?

Perhaps you feel that God is angry with you or displeased with you because you have succumbed to temptation. If an area of your life needs work, this does not mean God is angry with you. It means you have potential to grow and develop. God has more good things for you. He has blessings instead of condemnation. Your weight problem can become the impetus for a new goal. Instead of a noose around your neck, it can be a challenge in your side to move on with new ability through God's power. Victory over every problem, including overeating, is rightfully yours as a Christian person.

In the Old Testament God was displeased with the Israelites as they passed through the wilderness. He wasn't upset because they were in the wilderness, but because they assumed the wilderness as their only reality and left God out.

You also can be in the wilderness of life with seemingly no way out of temptation. Your appetite can seem a monster in your body. God wants to be more real to you than your appetite. You can confess, "God, I am stuck in the wilderness of my lust for food, but I choose to look up and grasp your supernatural power and ability. I choose you and the reality of knowing you, instead of eating."

Trust in God is a choice. When you come to Him and say, "God, I choose to trust you," God is then able to reveal himself to you in a new way. He is free to move in your life. You are more than thin when you commit yourself to trusting God's promises. It can actually be a blessing to feel desperate because that's when you are most ready to accept God's way to being all that you can be. A day will come when you say, "I am at last free to be *more* than the real me because I gave myself totally to God and His promises."

Pray: "Father, in the name of Jesus, I'm ready. I give myself to you right now because I will not be a victim of temptation any longer. You are faithful when I am not. Thank you that through all the tempting times you are with me. Thank you for your promises that challenge me with new goals and a new way of life as a thin person. In Jesus' name, amen."

three

A Greater Freedom

God is calling you into a deeper relationship with Him because He loves you. In your deeper relationship with the Lord, you will experience the victory of losing weight permanently. With your deeper commitment and closer relationship to God, you will discover greater freedom.

In order to handle freedom, you need to understand obedience. First Samuel 15:22 tells us, "Behold, to obey is better than sacrifice. . . ." In this use of "obey," the meaning is to hear, to hearken. Obeying and hearing are expressed by the same word in this instance. In other words, when God says, "Hear me," He is also saying, "Obey me by doing what I tell you." In order to obey God, we must develop the ability to hear what He says.

Two important features of the *Free To Be Thin* program are the keeping of a daily journal and being calorie accountable, which will be discussed in detail later. Now is a good time to begin your journal. It will provide you a record of God's guidance in your life, and help you evaluate what guidance you need.

One certain need is to hear Him concerning your goal weight. You also need His guidance concerning how many calories you should be eating daily. He is Lord of your body. He knows your frame and exactly how you should take care of it.

How Much Should I Weigh?

This is the question to ask the Lord. When you are committed to obeying Him, your listening is sharpened. You hear and obey as one action. Ask the Lord how much you should weigh. Ask Him what your calorie intake should be and then obey. When you ask intending to obey, you will receive.

God freely gives, so never be afraid to ask. The Lord wants to bless you. He wants to speak to you so that you can learn to obey Him. Your obedience in keeping a journal every day, for example, may sound about as much fun as vacuuming the rug. Maybe you find it difficult to answer letters, let alone write letters to yourself every day in your journal. But obedience is what you are seeking. The OV freedom plan includes being accountable for every calorie you put into your mouth. When you promise to obey the Lord, He promises to help you lose weight and a unique partnership is formed. He will support you with His strength. Through obedience you become part of God's beautiful plan for your ultimate best.

Helen wrote on her OV response sheet:

When I think of the relationship I have had with the Lord in losing weight and everything I've learned so far, I know that staying fat without Him would have been worse than any plague on earth. I have come to realize there is no free ride where obedience is concerned. My calorie limit is 1500 a day and I'm sticking to it!

Penny says:

I know I must learn to obey the Lord. I know that there is no turning back now and that God is telling me if I listen to Him and obey Him, I will achieve all He has promised me. I have 110 pounds to lose.

When the Lord Is Delighted

What does the Lord take great delight in? Obedience. Obedience is better than sacrifice. When we obey His voice we enter into a relationship with Him that is pure and unhindered. Have you ever watched a mother with her child? The mother asks, "Are you listening to me?" The child answers, "Sure, Mom," and then resumes what she was doing before. Delayed obedience does not delight the Lord, just as it does not delight a parent. To obey means you have heard and are responding immediately.

> **Obedience means hearing and responding to the Lord without delay.**

We can delight the Lord only when the Holy Spirit is dominating. It's virtually impossible to obey the Lord without the Holy Spirit, because you are naturally a self-absorbed person. To obey God means you are Holy-Spirit-absorbed.

The Change in Your Thoughts

When you obey the Lord with all your heart, your thoughts change. The thoughts that have been imprisoning you and keeping you fat will vanish and no longer hound you. The thoughts of food, eating for comfort, self-condemnation and guilt eventually come to an end when you learn obedience. You were once a slave to tempting thoughts, but no longer. Obedience to the Lord is your protection and your escape.

You may never have considered yourself a slave before, but that's what you are when you're consumed with thoughts of food. You're a slave when you eat without control. You're a slave when you eat all day long. You're a slave when you gorge one day and fast the next.

Meryl was a slave once. She explains:

> I would pick at a cake from the bottom, and I would eat
> around the edges of a meat loaf, and I would try to dis-
> guise the ice cream I ate by smoothing over the top. I was
> a slave to food. I felt so fat I wanted to die. I would eat
> until I hurt and all I could think of was eating more.
> There didn't seem to be any escape. I would eat so much
> I could only fall into bed and moan and groan. When I'd
> wake up I'd just eat again.

Meryl did not want to give up her own will when she
began attending a *Free To Be Thin* group. She pouted and
sulked like a child at the idea of obeying the Lord and
changing her habits.

Carla testifies:

> I'm 52 years old and I'm only learning now that I can
> control my eating habits—through the Lord! I've always
> done things my way and I've made a mess out of my whole
> life. I have been a glutton in every area of my life. I have
> been a glutton for attention, a glutton for food, a glutton
> for love, a glutton for things to go my own way. I have
> never been truly fulfilled. I have suffered with a temper
> and a critical spirit. I have never been truly happy with
> my life because I always felt there was something more,
> something better, something somebody else had that I
> should have.

Do you see what obedience to God can mean to you?
Both Meryl and Carla learned that obedience is not a bad
word. It doesn't mean restriction, it means freedom. Both
of these women have done more than lose weight—they've
gained new lives!

Connie wanted to be thin more than anything in the
world. She was a Christian without victory. She doubted
herself, doubted life and doubted there would be any help
for her.

Then one day she said yes to Jesus. She prayed quietly
and humbly with the girls in her group. "Jesus, I recognize
you are the Son of God. I also recognize I am a sinner.
Forgive me of my sin of overeating and cleanse me. I don't
want to be a victim of my own lusts. Fill me with your

Holy Spirit and make our wills one will. I choose to be obedient to you."

Connie has lost 52 pounds, but the best thing that has happened to her has not been the weight loss. She wrote in her journal, "I can honestly say I love obeying God. That's why I finally have victory over food." Connie is now free to be herself. Obedience brings freedom.

See the End Result

It isn't enough to say you're going to do something. Thinking about doing something will wax weary in time. You need to visualize your end result as you begin. Know that the end result is attainable and you can do it! See yourself free and thin. See your goal as already attained. Think of yourself as an obedient child of God. Hold onto your goal as a reality.

Joshua, in the Old Testament, was a great leader who was able to see the past, present and end result for his people. He constantly reminded the people from where they had come and to where they were heading. He reminded them it was God who had enabled them to escape captivity. He reinforced the truth that God was leading them and would continue to lead them. He reminded them of a sovereign God who loved them and demanded total obedience.

You once were a slave to food, as the Jews were slaves to Pharaoh. You were held captive by your own lusts, emotions and habits. Your loving heavenly Father led you out of destruction and bondage, and now you're on the road to the promised land (your end result). Remind yourself from where you came and to where you are going. See your goal as accomplished.

The Lord will accomplish what concerns me; Thy loving-kindness, O Lord, is everlasting: do not forsake the works of Thy hands.—Psalm 138:8

God has said that He will accomplish what concerns you and that His lovingkindness is everlasting. His word is true. Your words are true, too, when you are led by the Holy Spirit. You don't make false promises as you did before deciding to obey the Lord. You don't say things like, "Oh, Lord, I promise to be good no matter what. Never again as long as I live will I overeat."

The Lord loves your obedience. He loves your willing heart. Tell Him simply, "Lord, I choose to obey you."

. . . Then the Lord your God will restore you from captivity, and have compassion on you.—Deuteronomy 30:3a

Out of Captivity

You've been a captive of your eating habits, and God is now promising a way out. He wants to restore you and show you His compassion. Deuteronomy 30:5 promises, "And the Lord your God will bring you into the land which your fathers possessed, and you shall possess it; and He will prosper you and multiply you more than your fathers." God is going to do a wonderful work and prosper your weight-loss efforts. Losing weight is a goal you and He have together. He restores your entire being from captivity. You love the Lord your God, not your diet, and God prospers you in all you do. You'll be successful when you obey Jesus with your calorie account sheet as well as your heart and soul. Go back to the book, *Free To Be Thin*, and review how to set your calorie limit and find your goal weight.

When you choose obedience, be open to the Lord's guidance in what to eat and what not to eat. His guidance won't be too hard for you to follow. *"For this commandment which I command you today is not too difficult for you, nor is it out of reach"* (Deut. 30:11).

When you do not obey God, it may be you are not aware of God's will for you. It may be you haven't discovered how wonderful and exciting His plan for your life is. You may know only in part, with no vision of the end result. If you are still binging, God wants to deliver you from that captivity. You have a choice between life and death, the blessing and the curse. The *Free To Be Thin* person chooses *life*.

Jesus is our example of obedience, the way of choosing life. He shows us the way of obedience and He shows us it is possible.

Here is an assignment: Remembering that obey means to listen and then respond in action, write in your journal the ways you have positively responded to God (in action) in the past.

Listening to the Voice of the Lord

But this thing I did command them: Listen to and obey my voice, and I will be your God, and you shall be my people; and walk in the whole way that I command you, that it may be well with you.—Jeremiah 7:23, Amp.

In order for you to obey God's voice, remove those things that muffle His voice. You can't obey unless you hear. Learning how to listen to God is one of the most magnificent experiences you can have. When you go to Him and vent your problems, it is only fair to give Him equal time and listen to His advice.

His advice will never lead you on a wrong path. One OV leader tells her group, "Obedience is always followed by joy." When you hear the Lord whisper gently, "Don't eat that food; it's too fattening," and you obey, you will sense joy and the peace of self-control.

One OV'er was in the supermarket standing before the array of baked goods. She was quite hungry and knew she could polish off a package of caramel Danish pastries on the way home. Then she heard the Lord gently speaking to her spirit, "Don't do it." She turned and walked to the produce department where she chose a bag of apples. As she pushed the shopping cart to her car, she praised God for the ability to obey.

Am I Demon Possessed?

Darlene once insisted she had an overeating demon obsessing her and that her fat problem was not her fault. She went to her minister for prayer to be delivered of the demon.

She asked the minister, "Am I demon possessed?"

He told her, "The Lord loves you, Darlene, exactly as you are."

Darlene protested. "That can't be. I'm certain I'm demon possessed because I can't stop eating. Get rid of the demon for me and I'll be thin."

The minister shook his head, "Darlene, I do not sense a demon. I sense the love of God for you and I also sense some disobedience."

Darlene was outraged. "Disobedience! How can I obey when I can't help myself? I need deliverance. I just know my problem is because of something outside my control."

"You need the Lord Jesus and you need to obey His Word."

Darlene did change. The minister recommended she join an OV group, and in three months she lost 27 pounds and gained a new outlook on life as well. Darlene discovered there were no shortcuts and there were no excuses she could hide behind. She shakes her head when she remembers how she preferred the idea of being demon possessed over obedience to God.

The Scriptures say the Lord will write His law on your heart and mind. The change in your life comes from your heart and your mind. You must consciously choose to obey. It sometimes is not easy to humble yourself to walk in obedience. There may be times when you will not be willing to leave the table still hungry, but you will be willing to obey anyhow. There may be times when you aren't willing to refuse something fattening, but if you are willing to obey, you will be safe. There may be times when you are not willing to stay out of the kitchen when bored, but if you are willing to obey, you will be safe.

God is on your side. The Bible tells of an inner conflict between the spirit and the flesh. Galatians 5:17 says, "For the flesh sets its desire against the Spirit, and the Spirit against the flesh; for these are in opposition to one another, so that you may not do the things that you please." Obedience will help you overcome your overeating behavior, which is a work of the flesh. You were called to freedom, not captivity.

Once you are exposed to truth, you will never be able to be happy without its influencing all your decisions in life. Once God reveals to you that you are a sinner in need of His grace, you will never be happy until you act on that truth. Once He reveals to you that you can be free forever in Christ Jesus, living an abundant, happy and fulfilled life, you will never be satisfied until you experience the fulfillment of His promises.

Reasons for Disobedience

In a survey taken recently, over 200 people were asked, "Why do you overeat?" Out of all the answers, not one person said "hunger." The main reasons for overeating are anger, worry and fear.

Anger. Psalm 37:7–8 reads, "Rest in the Lord and wait patiently for Him. . . . Cease from anger, and forsake wrath. . . ." Anger can be deadly. If you suppress anger, you may run to food to help you feel better. Ulcers, headaches, backaches, insomnia, nervousness, and overeating are some of the consequences you may suffer when you do not deal with anger.

The above scripture tells us clearly to rest in the Lord. The Scriptures say be still, and though it may sound impossible, you can do it. It takes concentration and hard work to rest in the Lord. You cannot rest and harbor anger.

Confess your angry feelings to the Lord. Allow Him to heal you. As long as you hang on to the angry feelings and refuse to confess them, you may overeat, even binge. Tell the Lord, "I'm angry and I'm going to release the angry feelings to you because you know what to do with them. I confess anger to you and ask you to deliver me from harboring such feelings. Teach me to rest in you."

Worry. Ellen wrote on her OV response sheet:

> I know that worry has led into physical problems like my chronic upset stomach, my headaches and inability to sleep. I was always depressed and my appetite was and is still enormous. No matter what I worried about in the past I wanted to eat. Now I see that worry is a sin because worry is an expression of doubt in God's ability to take care of me.

Trust is the antidote for worry. *"Casting all your care upon him; for he careth for you"* (1 Pet. 5:7, KJV). God does the caring and He will work in your heart to help you change if you will let Him.

Philippians 4:6 says, *"Be anxious for nothing, but in everything by prayer and supplication with thanksgiving let your requests be made known to God."*

The command is "Be anxious for nothing," and the way to obey the command is: "In everything by prayer and supplication with thanksgiving let your requests be made known to God."

Think of the ways that God has already freed you. Be aware that your mind will deceive you if you allow yourself to complain. Bitterness is a deadly attack of the enemy, no matter how justified you think it may be. The Israelites nearly destroyed themselves by bitterness and worry. Joshua had to remind them God was on their side!

Fear. Fear is another one of your enemies. When fear is allowed to run loose in your life and do as it pleases, it stymies your thinking; causes your heart to palpitate; causes nausea, weakness and any variety of infirmities, including overeating.

Second Chronicles 20:17 says, ". . . Do not *fear* or be dismayed." The Lord is with you in every battle, especially the battle against your mind. When you grasp this truth you can give the problem to the Lord. Then you can face the problem with the assurance of His presence and power working in your behalf. Confusion and defeat come when you try to face the problem before you give it in surrender to God.

> **First face God with the problem,
> then face the problem with God.**

Accepting the Challenge

Read Philippians 2. Hold fast the Word of life. Prove yourself "blameless and innocent . . . in the midst of a crooked and perverse generation." Be a "light in the world." "Hold fast the word of life." Accept this challenge. A new desire for and level of obedience will spring up in your heart as you take a fresh attitude toward the commitment you made to the Lord at the beginning of this book. You can now say along with Jesus in Hebrews 10:9, "Behold, I have come to do Thy will."

The Bible says Abraham lived by faith as an alien in the land of promise. You can live by faith, learning obedience daily. As you consider your progress, think of it as a journey you have taken under the direction of the Lord Jesus. He is guiding you and showing you the way, just as He guided Abraham. He is protecting you and He is changing you. He is teaching you to be strong and to stand against temptation.

There is a big difference between obeying God and obeying a weight-loss program. The Bible does not say you can take Jean Nidetch or Nathan Pritikin or Neva Coyle with you when you stand before God on the day of judgment. When God looks at your life, He is not going to say to someone standing next to you, "How did she do?" He will ask *you*, and you will not be able to say, "If you want to know about my life, ask Neva."

The day will come when you will no longer need to count calories. That day will not come until you learn full obedience. The Lord will lead you through one discipline at a time, and that is why it is important to allow Him to do a full work in you each step of the way.

An Obedience Prayer

I will bless you, Lord, at all times,
Your praise is always in my mouth,
I sought you, Lord, and you answered me.
You delivered me from all my fears.
I have tasted of you and your ways, Lord, and
I know you are good.
I am blessed because I take refuge in you.
In you there is no want.
I seek you, Lord, and am not in want of any good thing.
I know your eyes are toward me, and
Your ears are open to my cry.
When I cry, you hear me, Lord,
And you deliver me out of all my troubles.
You have been near to me when I have been broken-
    hearted,
And you have saved me when I have been crushed in
    spirit.

Thank you, Father, for delivering me out of all
The afflictions I have experienced. You redeem my soul;
And because I take refuge in you, Lord, I will not be
    condemned.
Thank you, Father. Amen!

Psalm 34, paraphrased

four

A Place to Hide

The Fears of the Fat Person

Have you ever been so frightened you thought you were going to fall into little pieces all over the floor? That's how one OV'er described her past bouts with fear: "There are times I just don't think I can go on," she writes. "It's like I can't live and I can't die."

There are many fears the overeater experiences. She fears losing, missing out, and not getting enough to eat. The feeling is devastating.

You need two things in order to know you are secure in your commitment to be free to be thin: grace and peace.

2 Peter 1:2 says: *"Grace and peace be multiplied unto you through the knowledge of God, and of Jesus our Lord"* (KJV).

Grace is God's favor.

Peace is perfect well-being; all necessary good, all spiritual prosperity; and freedom from fears, agitating passions, and moral conflict.

The fears that plague the overeater are many. The fear of being hungry is a familiar one. Think of the time you have awakened in the middle of the night, and before going

45

back to bed, stopped at the cookie jar or freezer (home of the ice cream genie).

Fear need not be your master anymore. The lady who described her fear as "falling into little bits and pieces" read 1 Peter 1:2 and began to question why she had allowed herself to become a victim of fear.

God promises us spiritual prosperity. Depression, defeat and fear do not equal spiritual prosperity. Falling to pieces doesn't sound like prosperity of any kind.

The overeater's fear that there won't be enough food arises from insecurity. All insecurity can be traced to the lack of grace and peace being multiplied to us through the knowledge of God and Jesus our Lord. Some overeaters believe falsely that hunger is excruciating pain. They believe hunger is as bad as being terribly ill or dying. They view hunger as painful and morbidly unpleasant. Hunger seems cruel, unfair, excruciating, even indecent.

Another fear rises when the person nears the desired goal. An overeater starts to panic as she nears her goal weight. In the beginning she had to struggle with the fear that maybe she won't be able to maintain the goal. (We will discuss this in greater detail in Chapter 16.)

If the Lord is directing your eating program, He isn't going to allow terrible things to happen to you. He has promised spiritual prosperity. Psalm 138:8 promises: *"The Lord will accomplish what concerns me; Thy lovingkindness, O Lord, is everlasting; do not forsake the works of Thy hands."*

You can turn that promise into a prayer! "Thank you, Lord, for promising to accomplish that which concerns me. These are the things that concern me. . . (tell Him: Lord, I'm afraid once I reach my goal weight, I won't be able to keep it. I'm afraid of my appetite. . .)."

When you have open communication with the Lord, you won't harbor fears in your heart. You won't allow them to fester and ferment in your mind. Give them to

Him. God knows how to handle fear. His perfect love casts out fear and you will be able to look at yourself in the light of truth. It is true that you can't really trust yourself. But you can trust God.

God accomplishes what concerns you because He is intimately involved with you. There's security in that truth. It's the security you have longed for and have tried to find in eating. You never have found security in food, and you never will. But you can live free to be thin, with grace and peace multiplied within you and all around you. You can experience the Lord accomplishing that which concerns you, including your weight loss.

Fear of Pride

Some overeaters become insecure thinking they will become proud. One OV'er writes, "I always made excuses for my overweight because I told myself if I were thin, I'd be beautiful and then I'd be proud. I thought I'd probably get real carnal and go away from God if I looked too good."

What is in your heart will come out whether you are fat or thin. If you are going to fall from God, you don't have to lose weight to do it; you'll do it as a fat person. Refusal to exercise discipline and godly obedience is a most miserable form of pride. It's far more humbling to deny yourself your ungodly passion for eating than it is to remain fat and unhealthy.

An antidote for pride is firsthand observation of the miracles of God. You begin to see His magnificence. When you see Him for who He is, you can see yourself for who you are. You lose pride in your awareness of Him. You take your rightful place before Him as His worshiper and child. You cannot say He is almighty and glorious, and at the same time you are mighty and glorious. Praise to the Lord excludes praise of self.

There is immense security in giving the Lord every

victory. For example, if you start your *Free To Be Thin* program today, when you go to bed tonight thank God for the victory you had over your eating today. Give Him that victory as a gift. Tell Him, "Here, Lord, is the victory I experienced today by not overeating. I refused to snack before bed. I counted my calories faithfully. I obeyed you. I wrote in my journal. These are the victories for which I praise you." Your pride will go out the window along with your fat.

Emotional Eating

Have you ever eaten when angry? Depressed? Lonely? Insulted? One man admits coming home and eating an entire pecan pie after having an argument with a neighbor. Another man reveals he ate three dinners in three different restaurants when feeling lonely during a business trip away from his family. He came back to his hotel room miserably stuffed, and certainly not feeling secure or good about himself.

The Apostle Peter writes, *"His divine power has granted to us everything pertaining to life and godliness, through the true knowledge of Him who called us by His own glory and excellence"* (2 Pet. 1:3). *His* power *has* been given you. This is past tense. Power is already given to you for a life of godliness. If you *try* to live a godly life, working at being godly and good, you may fail. But if you pursue Jesus, you will gain godliness.

Talk to Him, confide in Him, be honest with Him. You will find yourself drawn to Him and pulled into Him as a moth into a cocoon. You'll be at home, secure, safe, because your life will be wrapped up in Him.

Without God you will not be secure no matter how you try to fill your life. If food won't satisfy you, neither will any external comforter. You won't feel secure with money, friends, job, position, accomplishments, abilities, or even your own good works. How many people do you know who spend their lives running around doing good for people, but are not secure? They're like flies buzzing around others' needs. "Oh, let me help," they buzz. But they are not helping out of the abundance of their contentment. They help because they think they should and because it makes them feel important and secure.

God has given you His power so you can be free of insecurities. You are free to make up your mind and live by that decision.

A Partaker of His Nature

Second Peter 1:4 says people can "*become partakers of the divine nature having escaped the corruption that is in the world by lust.*" It would be good to memorize that verse. Repeat it to yourself when you are feeling tempted, fearful, anxious or insecure. You are a partaker of God's nature. You can remain diligent because of His nature within you.

The verse says you have escaped corruption. Have you escaped your own corruption? Usually you are not worried about your friend down the block who is struggling with second helpings and midnight binges. Her corruption doesn't bother you. You may think, *Let them all get fat, so what?* But then your own personal enemy emerges, hungry and lacking motivation. And, if things didn't go too well today and you're feeling depressed and unloved, your enemy may lure your feet right toward the peanut butter and jelly.

This is the corruption you've got the power to escape from—your own corruption. It's at this precise time your homework will serve as armor. The preparations you made studying the Word, and your *Free To Be Thin* book, and keeping your journal and your calorie account sheet will now pay off.

You will not become secure by longing for security. You will not become godly by wishing you could be godly. Wishing and longing don't produce anything except more wishing and longing. Only the Word of God and communication with the Lord make the dramatic difference.

For we are His workmanship, created in Christ Jesus for good works, which God prepared beforehand, that we should walk in them.—Ephesians 2:10

Secure in Our Stronghold

The victory you will discover is what God has intended all along for you. You are reborn in Christ Jesus for victory, not oppression and defeat. If you begin to doubt that, look at Psalm 9:9 for a safe place to run: "The Lord also will be a stronghold for the oppressed. . . ."

Oppressed? Yes, that's you when hooked on food for security, when unhappily binging and purging, when centering every thought on eating or not eating.

The verse says the Lord also will be "a stronghold in times of trouble." Think of the many times you've eaten things you didn't want to eat; the many times you've eaten to please the one who prepared the food; the many times you've hated yourself for what you have eaten. You don't have to be fat to hate yourself for overeating and you don't have to be obese to be obsessed with food. If you are obsessed with food and overeating, you are oppressed; and the Lord wants to be your stronghold against that oppression.

When you're in trouble, He will be your stronghold, a place of safety. In Jesus you will be safe, secure, free from oppression and the barbed prongs of trouble.

A young wife from Los Angeles writes that she couldn't feed her family on low-calorie foods because they were too expensive. She says in her letter:

I gained weight right after I got married. Jim didn't make

a lot of money and I had to cook economically. That meant lots of starches and few fresh vegetables and fruits. With lettuce so high, I just couldn't afford it. So we ate tons of bread. I gained 25 pounds the first year we were married.

At the end of her letter she said:

Thank God I found *Free To Be Thin*. It changed my life. I was really dishonest with myself because even though I wouldn't pay a dollar for the lettuce, I thought nothing of paying a dollar for a package of cookies.

Was her problem the high cost of food? Is yours? If so, the Lord has promised to be a stronghold in times of high food costs.

Another woman writes, "My life has become a roller coaster. I've gained several pounds since I began the OV program. I feel like a 'squashed frog' whose lily pad has disappeared."

The Lord has promised to be a stronghold in times of roller coasters and missing lily pads. The "squashed frog" sounds like oppression. The Lord has promised to be a stronghold for the oppressed.

If you run to the Lord, He will be there. *"The Lord is good, a stronghold in the day of trouble, and He knows those who take refuge in Him"* (Nah. 1:7).

When Do You Need a Stronghold?

In your journal, on a separate sheet, make a list of the times when you most need a stronghold. A stronghold is a fenced place of protection, a fortress. It is a place where you are safe. Take your time as you make this list and be specific. If you need to elaborate a little, do it. Maybe you need a stronghold when your mother-in-law, the pastry chef, comes to town and she's brokenhearted if you don't eat her fabulous tarts and buns and biscuits.

Maybe your cousin Tony, the Italian wonder of the kitchen, has just called, insisting you "pop over for a little

bite." You're drooling before you hang up the receiver.
You can smell the tomato sauce and the cheeses. You know
if you step one foot into his kitchen, take one whiff of the
olfactory poetry he creates with food, you'll be hooked for
at least 2,000 calories and a guilt hangover big enough to
fill the Coliseum in Rome. The Lord is your stronghold in
times of Italian delights.

Aunt Louise, the thin one who can eat everything in
the known world and not gain an ounce, makes her own
ice cream. She calls to invite you over because she has
made a gallon of your favorite flavor. You become a wreck
of nerves at the thought. You can almost taste the ice
cream in your mouth. "Help!" you cry to Jesus as you run
toward Him. He is your stronghold in times of homemade
ice cream.

Make a list of your most difficult temptations. Add to
it; think about it. When is your most dangerous time of
day? When are you most likely to go bonkers at the thought
of cream cheese and crackers? When are you most tempted
to ravenously succumb to oppression, not caring what goes
into your mouth just as long as it's chewable and you can
swallow it?

A Journal Sample

I Need a Stronghold When:
- I go to my neighborhood Bible study and there, next
  to my Bible, is a plate of fresh, homemade doughnuts.
- At a ladies' luncheon they serve my favorite rich foods
  and I've paid for the meal, so tell myself I can't help
  it if there's nothing low-cal to eat.
- Cousin Tony calls at mealtime.
- The kids don't finish their meals and I hate to waste
  good food.
- I'm alone in the house with the Thanksgiving left-
  overs.

- Aunt Louise gets out the ice cream maker.
- I'm watching TV and the refrigerator is calling my name.

Stronghold means safety. How do you get to safety, to your stronghold? As *fast* as possible. The best way is through prayer. Your Daily Power Time is crucial if you're going to remain secure in your *Free To Be Thin* life. Here are some words from those who forgot where their place of security was:

- "I gained back eleven pounds and I'm wiped out. I hate myself."
- "It has been a real disaster for me these past months. I've been pigging out every day. Some days I don't even know what I've eaten. It's like I'm drunk."
- "I'm eating again and I'm gaining. I feel terrible."
- "I don't want to spread my gloom around, but these past weeks I've felt like a total failure. All I do is indulge. I eat every wrong food you can name and I can't stop."

These are the words of people who have lost sight of their security, their stronghold. Plan ahead for the day of temptation. Write your plan in your journal. Plan a godly, victorious response to temptation. See yourself facing a night alone at home with a loaf of bread on the kitchen counter, a pound of cheese in the refrigerator, peanut butter in the cupboard, and pizza in the freezer. Be ready to shout "Help!" and run into your stronghold.

Here's part of a letter from a woman who did not lose her security, but learned to find her stronghold daily: "My husband is the pastor of a church and at this time we are going through a trial. But since I have started the *Free To Be Thin* program, the Lord has begun a new work in me. Not only do the Scriptures you share deal with my eating, but every area of my life. I especially appreciate Philippians 1:6 and Psalm 138:8 (the Lord will perfect that which concerns me). I know He will answer the concerns of my heart regarding our church and family, and He will answer my concern to lose weight. I've already lost 13 pounds and I feel closer to the Lord than ever before in my life. I have learned how to run to Him as my safety from the temptation to feel sorry for myself and eat. I've learned to pray and read the Word."

A favorite portion of Scripture for this woman is Psalm 12:5:

> *Because of the devastation of the afflicted, because of the groaning of the needy, now I will arise, says the Lord; I will set him in the safety for which he longs.*

Carolyn tells her friends that the safety she always prays for is ability to handle social situations without being intimidated or defeated by the array of foods served. She continually has to prepare herself for those situations. She has to review the "I Need a Stronghold When . . ." pages in her journal.

Her solution to the Friendly Fattening Fellowship problem is to pray beforehand, "Lord, please allow something to be served that is nonfattening. If there is nothing there I should eat, I will understand you don't want me to eat."

Pray: "Lord Jesus, give us that special security that is ours in you. I choose now to personally find my safety in you. I run to you now as my stronghold. I run into the safety of your everlasting promises. I know that you hear my cry, that you are constantly listening, and that you care. In Jesus' name, amen."

five

What It Means to Be Desperate

An article in *The Los Angeles Times* tells of a 13-year-old boy who shot himself with his father's revolver. He is called "a lonely, overweight boy who isolated himself from friends and activities by eating and watching television." He weighed 255 pounds and was five foot six. He wrote a suicide note and the last words are, "In my heart I will take my TV with me. . . ."

We become desperate when we don't feel good about ourselves. One letter we received from a woman in Pennsylvania was cut in the shape of a circle. The lady writes:

This represents a very large and fat Christian (five foot six, 310 pounds). I just started reading *Free To Be Thin* as I am desperate. I know my overeating is sin and only Jesus can help me. [Signed] A very fat person.

A lady in Memphis writes:

Now I weigh 180 pounds. I never thought I would let myself go this far. I have really been totally out of control. My life is really at a low point. I have never been a very outgoing person, and now that I am so fat again I am avoiding almost all social situations. I don't want to be a recluse all my life. Please pray for me. I just want to experience wholeness in my life. . . ."

We receive thousands of letters from people all over

the world, crying in desperation. A lady in New York writes:

> I have read through *Free To Be Thin* every day for the last 14 days. It has given me the hope and opportunity of victory I didn't think would ever be possible. I have tried everything from heavy doses of amphetamines . . . to liquid protein and Dr. Atkins. I have never stayed thin nor kept the weight off.

The desperation takes on new character when we read words such as these from a woman in Texas: "I don't want to continue to be the jolly, fat woman in every group. I want to be the woman God would have me be."

A housewife in Michigan writes these heartrending words to Overeaters Victorious as her last hope:

> I am unhappy in my fat and I cry all the time. I just can't stop eating, though. Every day I vow, "This is the day I'm going to start dieting," and every day I blow it. My tears are filled with helplessness and frustration.

Each person who has battled with overeating understands. Another woman admits:

> There have been many times when I have sought the Lord with bitter tears concerning my weight. It has been an area in my life that I thought I could never get a handle on. Oh, yes, I've cried and cried.

"O Lord, give heed to my cry. . ." (Ps. 17:1b). In this chapter we are going to talk about our tears. It's important to know the kinds of tears we cry, for all tears aren't the same. The woman we just mentioned cried in general to nobody in particular. She simply felt bad and cried. Nothing uncommon about that.

There's a huge difference between crying your heart out when you feel bad and explicitly crying your heart out to Jesus. The first kind of tears go nowhere. They drip off the cheeks and dry up somewhere on the floor or in the wind. The second kind of tears catapult their way to the Master's love-heart where they become priority business to Him. These tears are written of in Psalm 107:6: *"They cried out to the Lord in their trouble; He delivered them out of their distresses."*

Give your tears to the Lord. Don't allow yourself to sit sorrowfully alone in your distress. Get up and cry to the Lord. He knows what to do with the trouble you're crying over. He knows how to deliver you. That's His business.

You Are Not Alone

When David wrote, "Lord, give heed to my cry" in Psalm 17, he was desperately telling God, "Listen to me! Listen to the hurt in my heart." That's exactly what you and I must do. A cry can be defined as uttering a loud sound. It is weeping, pleading, uttering a call characteristic of a child in trouble or a bird with a broken wing. David, a chosen servant of God, lived long before you and me, and spent much of his life crying to the Lord. You are not alone. David released his hurts and feelings of isolation by crying to the Lord. So can you.

David also cried to the Lord when he thanked Him. He cried in pain and he cried in thanksgiving. He was a man of tears, and not all of them sorrowful. "Weeping may endure for a night, but joy cometh in the morning," the Bible tells us in Psalm 30:5 (KJV). If you sit in your living room feeling sorry for yourself hoping God will eavesdrop on your thoughts, your tears aren't going to go into your "joy in the morning" account. Go ahead and be miserable tonight, as David was, but know that those tears, if given to Jesus, result in joy in the morning. He provides an escape, remember? He answers, He hears and He cares.

Judy writes:

> I started attending the *Free To Be Thin* class. I was so hungry to feel God's love. I had never felt good about myself. I blamed my husband for my feelings of failure, and I blamed my church for my lack of spiritual growth.

I cried unto the Lord and He began to minister to me. The weight started to melt off. By August I had lost 20 pounds. By December I had lost 40 more pounds. I now weigh the same as when I was in the ninth grade. I was healed of being overweight! Just like when being sick, I was healed of a lifetime problem of being a thin person trapped in a fat body. My tears are of joy now.

Approximately 50 million people in North America are trying to lose weight this very moment. It is estimated there are 40 million people in the United States alone who are 10% to 20% above their recommended weight. Yet, with all of the weight-loss plans, programs, pills, powders and contrivances, American people are *gaining* weight, not losing it. The National Center for Health Statistics says men weigh nine pounds more than the 1960 male average and women weigh nearly thirteen pounds more than the female average of a decade ago.

Adult Americans' stored fat amounts to 2.3 trillion pounds, and of the 10 million Americans who are trying to reduce that statistic today, only 7% succeed in reaching their goal weight. If that isn't enough to draw a tear or two, consider this: less than 2% maintain their goal weight for one whole year and less than 1% maintain their goal weight for the rest of their lives.

You are not alone in your battle. We believe this book will help you win your battle. You can be one of the people in the 1% lifetime maintenance category. You can because you are not alone: God is right there at your side to help you.

Crying to the Lord comes from an awareness of your need. Psalm 3:4 tells us how David cried to the Lord.

But Thou, O Lord, art a shield about me, My glory, and the One who lifts my head. I was crying to the Lord with my voice, and He answered me from His holy mountain.

When David verbalized his need to God, God answered. David didn't waste time crying on other people's shoulders, he cried to God. He went to the one in charge, to the Creator.

If you're in trouble, cry to God, not your friends. One woman we know called everyone in her address book to tell them her troubles when she was upset. God was the last one she talked to. Then she learned to cry to the Lord. She discovered if David could cry his heart out about his troubles to God, she could too.

Psalm 107:5–9 tells us:

Hungry and thirsty they fainted; their life was near being extinguished. [Sound familiar when you're trying to lose weight?] *They cried to the Lord in their trouble, and He delivered them out of their distresses.* (Amp.)

Free To Be Thinners need to learn how to cry to the Lord when losing weight. Sometimes you'll feel hungry and thirsty. How are you going to handle feeling hungry? What will you do when you get up from the table after eating, still feeling hungry? You tell yourself, "So this is what it feels like when a person is losing weight!"

He led them forth by the straight and right way [your new calorie account sheet], *that . . . they might establish their homes* [stability through obedience]. *Oh, that men would praise* [and confess to] *the Lord His goodness and loving-kindness, and His wonderful works to the children of men!*—Psalm 107:7–8, Amp.

God will help you achieve a new, healthy body.

You can experience hunger and not necessarily starve to death. You must talk to yourself as a parent talks to a child. "No, self, you aren't going to die without that second helping. You may not have any more to eat right now. You may eat again at mealtime."

God is establishing you with strength by His goodness and loving-kindness. You are His wonderful work. "For He satisfies the longing soul, and fills the hungry soul with good." There's your dessert right there. What could be tastier and more wonderful than being filled with goodness?

A New Way of Talking to Yourself

Dialogue with yourself using statements like these:

"It's amazing how fast time goes by. I'll be having my next meal before I know it. I cannot eat now, no, not even one more bite."

"I won't die of hunger just because other people are eating rich, fattening foods and I'm not."

"I can go without. I really can."

"So this is how it feels to lose weight. What a wonderful feeling!"

"Praise the Lord, I have His power to have power over myself."

"I will not eat _____(fill in the blank). I will cry unto the Lord to help me not eat it."

"I cry unto the Lord and He delivers me out of my distresses."

"Lord, take my 'I can'ts' and turn them into 'I wills.' "

"This is a *quid pro quo* arrangement—something for something. I cry and the Lord delivers. I give Him my body and He blesses it. I commit myself to my *Free To Be Thin* program and He sees to it the weight comes off."

"I resist the temptation to attempt a radical diet plan in which I eat less than I should, or not eat at all. There are no shortcuts to permanent weight loss."

"I commit myself to losing weight *permanently*. I commit myself to staying thin. I commit myself to my body's future."

"I am going to be honest with myself and with God. I am going to stop lying about my weight and about what I eat."

Being Honest with Yourself

Crying to the Lord will help you accept the truth about your eating behavior. You can dare to admit what you've been afraid to face because you can immediately run to Jesus about it and pour it all out to Him. You can dare to look in the mirror and face the fact that you really are as fat as you look. You can look at yourself and admit the truth, instead of offering feeble excuses such as, "I'm too short to wear this dress the way it ought to be worn," or "Short people always look heavier than they really are." God knows you're short and He knows how much you weigh and ought to weigh. Talk to Him about it. Tell it like it is.

Marie Chapian had her day of reckoning. In her book, *Fun To Be Fit*, she writes, "What a horrible shock it was to discover the mirror I was looking in wasn't a trick mirror distorting my thin image. The pudgy person staring wide-eyed back at me was none other than myself. 'But I'm fat!' I gasped. 'How can this be? I don't feel fat. I feel athletic and—*short*.'" This painful experience inspired a new commitment to health and fitness. It catapulted her into a renewed *Free To Be Thin* commitment and the development of her "Blessercize" program.

When you're free to be thin, less is more.

Psalm 17:1 says, "Give ear to my prayer, which is not from deceitful lips." To become thin, you must become honest. You may be tearfully pleading with God to help you lose weight, yet chomping on huge samples of the meal you're cooking. Later you sit down to your weight-loss portion of cottage cheese and salad, feeling very self-righteous. Afterward you clean up Junior's half-eaten pumpkin pie and while putting away the dishes, you spot two uneaten dinner rolls and nibble them, one tiny bite after another, as though taking smaller bits removes calories. Later that evening when friends drop by with ice cream and cake, you tell yourself, "Well, I can eat a big portion because all I had for dinner was that little bit of cottage cheese and a salad."

Have you ever hidden the truth about how much you really weigh? Is the weight on your driver's license true? A physican who specializes in eating disorders in Minneapolis completed a study in which people were put on a diet and told to write down everything they ate during the week. The people did as instructed, but when they returned to the next meeting, they hadn't lost weight.

The same people were then placed in a controlled situation for one week and given the exact diet they had written on their sheets. The most amazing thing happened—they lost weight.

Crying to the Lord makes you honest. "Please make me honest" should be included in your new dialogue with the Lord. "Help me be honest about myself. Help me face the truth and not run from it or deny it."

You may discover you really *are* as fat as you look, that you really *are* eating too much. Instead of telling yourself, "I'm fat because of my metabolism," you can admit the truth: "I eat too much." Crying to the Lord in honesty will help clear the road between your present weight and your goal weight.

Your attitudes will change with your new freedom to cry to the Lord. You will discover a change in yourself, not only toward food and your body, but toward God, your family, friends, work and co-workers.

Your newfound freedom to cry to the Lord will liberate other areas of your life. Where you once may have been judgmental and hard, you will find yourself more compassionate and understanding. Where you once may have been jealous and prone to backbiting, you will find yourself admiring and generous.

It's okay to cry to the Lord about *everything*. He is never intimidated by your cries. He is never troubled by your troubles. He is compassionate and wise and powerful. God never gets depressed because you are. "Let not your heart be troubled, neither let it be afraid" are the words of an untroubled God.

Then they cried out to the Lord in their trouble; He delivered them out of their distresses.—Psalm 107:6

Whatever distresses you today, tomorrow, next week, whenever and whatever, cry to the Lord with them. Crying can be with or without tears. Men don't like to cry tears because they have been taught tears are sissy stuff, less than masculine. "Only girls cry," a ten-year-old boy agonized to his teacher as he lay on the ski slope with a broken leg. Crying doesn't mean tears. That little boy was crying without tears. You can cry with your voice, with your whole self, and not shed one tear. Make sounds, verbalize, *tell* the Lord the cry of your heart. Crying is telling. Crying to the Lord is telling Him all.

It may not be honest to tell Him, "Lord, I can't stop eating." When you're being honest, you realize what you are really trying to say is, "Lord, I *won't* stop eating." He delivers you out of your distress so you can say, "Lord, I *will* stop eating—with your help."

Pray: "Thank you, Lord, that you deliver me out of my distress when I cry to you. Just now, in the name of Jesus, I'm crying to you. I confess the food I have eaten has held me in bondage. I confess when I have attended social activities I've eaten too much and been ashamed. I confess I have abused birthdays and the holidays of Thanksgiving and Christmas. I have used special occasions as a reason to binge and gorge myself. I confess my feelings of failure and defeat. Your Word says you are delivering me out of these distresses, and I thank you. I receive the ability to be a victorious eater right now. In Jesus' name, amen."

The Freedom of Discipline

Discipline Is Not a Nasty Word

"When I joined Overeaters Victorious I weighed 180 pounds," a Wisconsin coed testifies. "Tonight I weigh 142 and have 10 more pounds to lose to reach my goal weight. These last pounds are very difficult because I find that I still have to learn the same lessons over and over again. I want to eat when I want to eat, and I want to eat anything that appeals to me. Sometimes I hate discipline."

Discipline can appear to be no fun, representing pain and self-denial. "How can I be disciplined about my eating?" this student asks helplessly. "I have very few rewards in my life and the best thing I have is food. Eating is positively the only reward in my life. How am I supposed to deny myself this? You tell me."

Does discipline sound like a nasty word to you?

In some Bible versions the word discipline is translated punishment. Most people hate restriction in their lives. It's like punishment. But the Word of God says:

Do not regard lightly the discipline of the Lord, nor faint when you are reproved by Him; for those whom the Lord loves He disciplines.—Hebrews 12:5, 6a

Discipline is a nasty word to many people because they

expect God to discipline the way they discipline children—scream at them, take something away, send them to their room without supper, dock their allowance, storm out, physically abuse them. In other words, most people expect God to hurt them the way a bullying parent would hurt a child.

Hebrews 12 says God will discipline you, but "the kindness of God leads you to repentance" (Rom. 2:4). Do you expect God to slap that brownie out of your hand and give you a permanent toothache for going off your diet? How many times have you gone off your diet and attributed to the judgment of God every bad thing that happened afterward?

The above college student tells how she binged on pizza and ice cream one Friday night. "God punished me for it later," she presumptuously explained, "because on Saturday I got a flat tire, a sore throat, and accidentally bounced a check."

Her OV counselor questioned her: "Do you really believe God did all that to you?"

"Oh, yes, that's His way of making me pay for binging." How wrong she was.

God is not waiting behind the refrigerator for you to commit the sin of gluttony. He's not prowling around bakery entrances hoping you'll walk through so He can jump out and shout, "Fatty, fatty, two-by-four. . . !" He's not waiting for you to binge on pizza and ice cream so He can puncture a tire or give you a sore throat. He's not hiding in the kitchen to catch you dropping Oreos into your mouth. No, a voice is not going to boom from above, "Shame on you! I'll get you for that."

God will *not* say to you:

"You're a hopeless case."
"You ate what you shouldn't have, so I'm finished with you."

"I'm sick and tired of your problems."

"You're fat and you'll always be fat."

"That was your last chance."

"Don't bother me with your dumb questions like, 'Why is everything good fattening?'"

"Don't you ever speak to me like that again."

"If you ever behave like that in front of me again, I'm through with you."

"I'm sick of you and your empty promises."

"You say one thing but you do another. How much can I take?"

"I'm at the end of my rope with you. You'll just never change."

"This relationship is completely one-sided."

"Why, oh, why, did I ever trust you?"

"You know what you are? A human yo-yo, that's what. Lose ten pounds, gain back twelve. I don't want to hear about your desire to be thin. You never listen to me anyhow."

"If there's one thing I can't stand it's a failure."

God *does* say to you:

"Whom the Lord loves He disciplines" (Heb. 12:6).

"It is for discipline that you endure. . ." (Heb. 12:7).

"Therefore, strengthen the hands that are weak and the knees that are feeble" (Heb. 12:12).

"I will never desert you, nor will I ever forsake you" (Heb. 13:5).

"There is therefore now no condemnation for those who are in Christ Jesus" (Rom. 8:1).

Spiritual Running

It is time now in your *Free To Be Thin* commitment to move into a deeper, closer relationship to God in the area of weight control. First Corinthians 9:24–27 asks, "*Do you*

*not know that those who run in a race all run, but only one
receives the prize?"* This is what you are doing when you
make your commitment to give God control of your body.
The verse concludes with, *"Run in such a way that you
may win."*

How many people start the dieting race and don't finish? When a woman commits herself to a weight-loss plan,
it's because she has hit rock bottom. She is limping at the
very end of the race. She is crying out to God for help.

"Do you not know that those who run in a race all run,
but only *one* receives the prize?" Only 1% maintain their
weight loss. This scripture says only a few win. You can
be one of them. You are on the side of the Lord Jesus
Christ. He is victorious and His victory and freedom are
within you. You can win because the victory is already
yours. You were created to run like a winner. You are free
to be thin!

When Are You a Non-Winner?

"Run in such a way that you may win" means to stop
running like a non-winner.

- You don't win when you buy fattening junk food for
  your cupboard and refrigerator shelves.
- You don't win when you blame somebody else for
  your overeating. Being angry at your spouse, boss or
  children is not an excuse to overeat.
- You don't win when you fail to prepare yourself for
  discipline at mealtimes.
- You don't win when you fail to make a commitment
  to yourself and the Lord to fulfill His plan for your
  life.
- You don't win when you tell yourself discipline is
  painful and unpleasant, instead of a joyful gift.

In order to stay out of those non-winning ranks, you
need to be aware of some sneaky enemies. One is buying
non-winning foods and the other is eating them. There are

certain restaurants you should avoid if you can't eat sensibly there. One OV'er told us she was practically "starving to death" and still not losing weight. When we questioned her, she told us she ate only one meal a day. Here's what she ate:

1 Big Mac	563 calories
1 vanilla shake	352 calories
1 large french fries	430 calories
1 apple pie	253 calories
Midafternoon: Pepsi (12 oz.)	160 calories
Late afternoon: Pepsi (12 oz.)	160 calories
Evening: 2 Pepsis (12 oz. each)	320 calories
TOTAL	2238 calories[1]

Awareness of the calories in what you eat will set you on the course of the winner. That lady was gaining weight, not losing it. She had no idea she was stuffing herself with 1,000 excess calories a day.

Choose Your Influences

Once you choose to run your race like a winner, you will not only become aware of what you are eating and how many calories you are consuming, you will become aware of your influences. What is your biggest influence? People. Be aware of whom and what you listen to. If your friends are encouraging you to remain overweight, know that a winner doesn't listen to non-winner advice.

Choose companions who will encourage you. If you need correcting or uplifting, be sure you have someone to call. This is the advantage of being in a *Free To Be Thin* group. There is always someone available to lift your spirit and encourage you.

A non-winning influence is someone who advises that

---

[1] Barbara Kraus, *Calories and Carbohydrates* (New American Library, 1983).

you are just fine the way you are, when you are not. Advice you don't need says, "God looks at the inward person. He doesn't care if you're fat or skinny."

God wants to be first in every area of your life. If He is not first in your eating, He wants to be. He is concerned that you win your race over your undisciplined appetites. He wants to empower you to win. *"Everyone who competes in the games exercises self-control in all things"* (1 Cor. 9:25). When you allow the Lord to discipline you, something amazing happens. You ask for discipline in your eating habits, but He touches more than your eating habits. There is a miraculous transformation in your inner heart attitude; self-control in all things becomes possible.

Others will notice the change and you will affect their lives, though this may take time. Thousands of letters received at the OV office tell how *Free To Be Thin* has not only changed their lives, but the lives of friends and family as well. One woman from Indiana writes:

> I went to my *Free To Be Thin* class faithfully every week and slowly my life began to change. I not only learned a new way of eating, I learned a new way of life. Then one day my teenage son asked me how come I was so different. My husband began paying me compliments and wanting to be with me more. My daughters and I, we weren't even on speaking terms, started to get close. Within four months I lost 22 pounds and my entire family came to Jesus. We're closer than we've ever been and I have totally changed. I'm a new person inside and out. My oldest son has lost seven pounds and even my husband has lost 12 pounds. Thank you, *Free To Be Thin*, and most of all, thank you, Jesus [Signed] Beth.

Connie, from New Hampshire, writes that she conquered anger and self-pity, and lost 32 pounds as well. Which is she most thankful for? "I'm most thankful," she writes, "for the influence I've had on my family and friends. They know I had to have supernatural help because I've never lost weight and kept it off before in my life. Furthermore, I was known for my bad temper and moodiness. Not anymore!"

This letter from Kathy in California touched our hearts. She writes:

> I have been overweight for the past 13 years. After *Free To Be Thin* I went from 142 pounds to 110 pounds (I'm five foot one). I am actually free from the bondage of overeating. I want you to know that I did not have to struggle to do this—it seemed effortless as I kept my eyes on the Lord. There was no doubt in my mind that the Lord was performing a miracle—doing something for me that I could not do for myself. I can say with certainty that I have never been happier or more full of joy. And the greatest thing is when people want to know about this change in my life and I am able to share what Jesus has done for me.

Free to Be Disciplined

When discipline enters your life, it will make you free. You will experience release and new ability through discipline. A housewife complains, "What a drag my life is. I have to make the beds, do the dishes, finish the laundry . . . it's endless. I hate it." She then discovers discipline and little by little her attitudes change. Discipline frees her. Instead of being unhappily trapped in housework, she is set free to love God, love herself and appreciate the work of her hands, whatever that work is.

> *All discipline for the moment seems not to be joyful but sorrowful; yet to those who have been trained by it, afterwards it yields the peaceful fruit of righteousness.*—Hebrews 12:11

If you're a student you can be free to finish your homework assignments, free to write the theme papers that are due, free to achieve your goals and earn the grades you want.

At the job you're free to succeed. You're free to get along with your boss and fellow employees, free to be the boss—a good one—free to prosper, free to win your race.

When you're free, you're happy. Discipline is no longer laborious because instead of being hindered by it, you're set free by it. You are free to do not only what you want, but also what you know you should. You are calorie accountable.

Discipline is like a fortified wall around a city. It protects you.

Gaining the Imperishable

Athletes exercise self-control in all things "to receive a perishable wreath, but we an imperishable" (1 Cor. 9:25). The weight-loss goal you have chosen is perishable, because your body is not eternal. But the work God is doing in your life as you lose weight is permanent—imperishable. Self-control and discipline will remain with you and be imperishable. You'll be stronger than ever before and your strength won't perish. As wonderful as your new thin body will be, your spirit will outlast it. You're a spiritual person first, a physical one second.

Goals

The Apostle Paul had a clear goal: *"Therefore I run in such a way, as not without aim; I box in such a way, as not beating the air"* (1 Cor. 9:26). What is your aim in losing weight? You need goals. Where are you going? Where have you been? Make your highest aim to be like Jesus in all things. Jesus never binged on junk food. He never had a food fettish. Allow God to build dignity and character within you so you can glorify Jesus.

If you are running in a race and don't know where you're going, you are really in trouble. You may be running backward and not know it. You may take a wrong turn on the course, you may pass the finish line, lose your way. It doesn't matter how great a runner you are. You could be an Olympic gold medalist, but if you don't know where you're running, you have lost the race before you have begun.

Run with an aim. Set goals. First, set short-range goals because these, in turn, lead to long-range goals. The Apostle Paul said he boxed "in such a way, as not . . . beating the air." Common sense tells you if you want to hit something, you don't want to waste strength punching the air. You don't spend your potential foolishly. You go after the goal.

Not "beating the air" when you are becoming free to be thin means you don't use your energy foolishly. You don't lose weight just for an upcoming wedding or high school reunion. You don't starve yourself and sweat in the sauna for 12 days to lose 10 pounds for a family portrait. That's being preoccupied with food. Not eating can be as bad as overeating.

Running with an aim means pursuing goals (read chap. four in *Free To Be Thin*). The Lord wants to help you set your goals. He knows your frame, your muscles, heart. He knows every cell. How much does *He* want you to weigh? Pray and ask Him to show you.

Usually you would choose to weigh less than what the Lord's will for you is. You may be hard on yourself but He isn't hard on you. One woman in an OV group announced at the first meeting she wanted to lose 50 pounds and weigh 106. She was five foot five and had a medium frame. After praying with a partner and listening for the Lord for a couple of weeks, she told her group, "The Lord told me to lose 36 pounds and weigh 120 for His glory. Praise the Lord, He spoke to me! I know He has definitely told me how much to weigh. He cares!" Six months later this same woman reached her goal and has stayed there.

It is important that you allow the Lord to speak to you. He has only the best in mind for you.

Pray: "Lord Jesus, I thank you for calling me to live a life of discipline. Forgive me for my past undiscipline and selfishness. I choose now to allow you to speak to me, help me, change me and guide me by your Word, the Scriptures. Thank you for loving me and for the promise of victory which you give freely to me when I choose your way and not my own. Thank you for telling me you will never leave me nor forsake me, because I need you. I commit myself to your discipline because your discipline is loving and good. In Jesus' name, amen."

seven

Discovering the Real You

When was the last time you looked in the mirror and said, "Hello there, me. Nice to see you"? Have you *ever* said, "When I look at me I look at a person I know very well and like very much"? If you're like most people, you haven't done either of the above. Overweight people in particular don't say many positive things to themselves about themselves.

How can you discover the honest-to-goodness real you? You spend more time with you than anyone else does, so why not invest some time in getting on intimate terms with yourself. Some people treat themselves as a distant relative, someone they are related to but rarely encounter personally. A conversation with a person who hasn't quite gotten to know herself might go like this:

"Would you like to go with me to the new department store at the mall and browse?"

"Oh, I don't know. . . ."

"Maybe you'd rather go for a walk in the neighborhood?"

"Well, whatever you want."

"How about taking a drive to the park and walking around the lake?"

"If you want to, it's okay with me."
"I would like to do what *you* want."
"It doesn't matter."
"But it matters to me. What would you like to do?"
"Whatever you say. . . ."

How passive can you get? Who are you and what do you want?

With a little effort you can discover yourself. You may be pleasantly surprised to learn what a wonderful person you've been missing out on. Instead of greeting yourself in the mirror with, "Hello, fat person. I feel sorry for you because nobody likes fat people" (unspoken in the past, but felt nonetheless), you can learn to say, "Hello there, me. I believe in you, and I believe you will reach the goal you've set before you. The Lord is your Shepherd; you shall not want."

Hearing God Speak to You

It is vital to the success of your weight loss that you allow the Lord to speak to you and that you hear His voice. How do you do this? Discipline is again the answer, because He speaks to you through His Word. The only way to hear Him speak to you through His Word is to schedule time for reading, studying and meditating on His Word. This is your Daily Power Time. A time of communication with the Lord is the first and most important requirement for your new life as a *Free To Be Thin* person.

Most of the people surveyed who have lost more than 30 pounds on the program say they preferred to have their devotional time with the Lord in the morning. Whatever time of day is best for you, *schedule* it. Don't rely upon the vague hope that you'll maybe have time later, maybe after lunch sometime before the kids get home from school, or after work. Something will invariably interrupt you. The telephone will ring, the doorbell will sound, the dog will tip over his water dish, you'll notice your philodendron needs watering, you'll remember you need to go to the bank, you'll see a friend and run outside to talk just for a moment—there's no end to what can interfere with your time with the Lord.

Set a time. This is the time that you give to God. It is a gift from you to Him, an offering. "Let each one do just as he has purposed in his heart; not grudgingly. . ." (2 Cor. 9:7). Your time with God is sacred and holy. It can be your excursion into glory each day if you let it be. This time set will result in an inner wealth you cannot begin to perceive now. Each week, month and year it gets better. ". . . he who sows sparingly shall also reap sparingly; and he who sows bountifully shall also reap bountifully" (2 Cor. 9:6).

Your Daily Journal

One of the most successful and exciting features of the OV program is the discipline of the daily journal. For the many thousands who have lost weight through this program, it has been a key to opening the way for victory and self-understanding.

Get a notebook and pen and keep them with your Bible. Buy a notebook in which you can make many entries. Choose one you like, that you'll enjoy writing in. A favorite notebook of many Free To Be Thinners is the *Free To Be Thin Daily Planner.* A small looseleaf notebook with tabs to separate subjects is also useful. A calorie-counting book is an inseparable part of your journal. You must know how many calories you are eating. The journal will show you why, how, where and when you are eating. You'll spot patterns and get at the roots of your behavior. You'll discover the answers the Lord has for you.

Record your Scripture verse for each day in your journal. Write down the thought the Lord is impressing on you, and what you are telling the Lord. A question you should answer at the end of a week is: What principles has the Lord taught me this week? How can I be more faithful next week? What changes am I seeing in my attitudes toward food, God and people?

Thousands of people have lost weight on the *Free To Be Thin* program and kept it off. Here are some comments by Free To Be Thinners regarding the discipline they've gained and what their journal has meant to them:

> I am more aware of my eating than ever before. It's shocking how ignorant I was about what went into my mouth. I'm counting calories and having more Bible study than ever in my life even though I was a Christian for 18 years.

> Because I have learned the discipline of keeping a daily journal, I think more about what I am doing. I also think more about God. I talk more about Him and what He's doing in my life. People listen to me. They know something special has happened to me.

> I feel better about myself and closer to God. I know He is with me and He cares.

> I never realized the Lord really cared about my overweight. I've always been fat and I never thought the Lord cared about how unhappy I was about it. He has shown me He cares. Each day He helps me and speaks to me through His Word about how much He cares.

> My journal shows me how much I've changed! The end is in sight! I've lost 36 pounds so far, but the best is how much I've changed inside.

> Over Christmas I blew it, but I looked over my journal and I can see why I did it. I could feel a terrible failure, but looking over my journal encourages me. I must not resort to guilt and more overeating. I've lost 27 pounds and have 25 more to go. I know the Lord will help me.

> Discipline has taught me not to let my body tell me what to do.

> My journal has personalized God to me. At first I didn't

know what to say every day because I was unaccustomed to being so personal with Him. I wanted to copy down other peoples' prayers and inspirational poems, but instead I had to write something from *my* heart, *my* feelings, *my* goals and desires. When I got to the part about writing down what He was saying to me, it was somewhat of a shock. It was so wonderful, I could hardly grasp it. God spoke to me! His Word spoke to me! Now I can write, "God told me today in the Scriptures . . ." and complete the sentence. It's wonderful.

I delight more in the Lord now. I see Him more clearly. I know Him better.

I feel much better about myself. I've learned how much He cares about me because I spend time with Him every day. I never used to be so consistent. I've lost 32 pounds, but the change in me personally is far greater than the weight loss.

I study the Word more intensely and feel I have a closer walk with the Lord. I know more about His will for my life. I know it is not His will I be fat and unhappy.

The Lord and I just keep getting closer and closer.

I'm much more aware of what has been going on inside me. I'm also much more grateful to the Lord because I've experienced His forgiveness and mercy. I've got it down in black and white.

My journal and counting calories has been like a security blanket. This week I ate in restaurants for *seven* meals. If I weren't committed to my journal and calorie account sheet, I would have blown it for sure. My daily Scripture verses held me up, strengthened me and kept me in God's will. I did not overeat and I drew closer to Jesus instead of away from Him.

Drinking was a problem with me but keeping a journal has made me see how rebellious and self-centered I've been. Now I know the Lord is with me and I'm on the right road with Him. I'm delivered from alcohol forever. I'm more yielded to God than I've ever been. Keeping my

journal and my daily time with Him has saved my life.
My friends all tell me I'm like a totally new person. I've
given up smoking, too, and I don't even miss it!

Jesus can do anything. He has shown me I can live a life
worthy of Him. My goal is to please Him in every way,
bearing fruit in every good work, growing in the knowledge of God. I can because He can. He can change me.

When I read Jesus' words to the crippled person, "Do you
want to be healed?" I knew He was speaking to me, too.
I couldn't put my problem off any longer. I had made too
many excuses to stay fat. "Yes, Lord, I want to be healed,"
is what I wrote in my journal. That was two months ago.
I've lost eleven pounds and I can honestly say it seems
like the pounds just melted off. I *want* to be healed.

My daily study of the Word is like my food. I feast on it
hungrily and take long notes for my journal. It's my most
special time of the day.

I have learned to be consistent with my Daily Power Time,
something I never was before.

I can follow good eating habits until the middle of the
afternoon; then I tend to start snacking and it is hard to
find a stopping place. One thing that has happened to me
is that when I have my Daily Power Time in the morning
and I take time to write in my journal, I have strength
for the hard time of temptation in the afternoon. I don't
succumb because I remember what the Lord told me
through His Word that morning.

I have come to realize that I have a responsibility to be
obedient and do my part, which I've never done before. I
realize that I can be disciplined, but I must work to make
it come out in my life.

My journal keeps me coming to God and gives me a chance
to trust Him and see Him at work in my life.

My journal keeps me in the Word and keeps me bound to
my commitment to Him.

A Truth a Day Keeps the Devil Away

Allow God to impress one powerful truth on you each day. Walk in that truth and by the end of seven days you will have seven profound truths you've learned and experienced. At the end of the year, you'll have learned 365 truths from God through His Word. Just one truth a day will change your life because you're not just acknowledging and reciting the truth, you're *experiencing* it.

You have the power of God within you to change yourself. Focus in on the *one* truth God is teaching you each day. In your journal write what's in your heart about the verse. Write what you are telling the Lord, the deepest cry of your heart, the deepest need, the deepest joy, the deepest praise; get it all down on the paper. Don't worry about anyone else reading your private notes. They are not for any eyes but yours and the Lord's. Express your thoughts and feelings. They are important today and they will be important to review later.

Your time alone with God is your permanent daily commitment. The Lord Jesus has promised to be your teacher, friend and guide. His voice is not too hard to hear. His instruction is not too difficult to understand. Trust Him to speak to you and help you discover yourself.

B.C.

I knew loneliness
before.
Barren, scalding
loneliness.
When scorpions devoured the days
and the nights
when time
screamed by
in heaps of rubbish
on the way to the
dump.
When my life
lay gnarled and severed
in a bag of
rags.
I knew loneliness
before.

I knew loneliness when
I ached
so passionately
to mean a little something
to
    someone.

But now
let me tell you,
the crushing weight
of loneliness
will never touch my life
        again
because the Master Jesus
has claimed me for His
own.

I am His
    someone.

—Marie Chapian[1]

---

[1]*City Psalms*, Moody Press 1971.

eight

Rebuilding Your Temple

Jeff says:

Last year I weighed 330 pounds. The year before that I weighed 370 pounds. The weight was destroying my back and I was having chest pains which scared the daylights out of me. The doctor told me I had to lose weight, so I tried and tried and after 13 months I had only lost 40 pounds. I was discouraged and resentful.

I had so many defenses built up, so much resentment and distrust I didn't even want to go outside. I told my wife, "I'm not going to go out because people will talk about me. They'll laugh or stare." She dragged me to a *Free To Be Thin* meeting. I went kicking and screaming in protest because I had tried everything in the past to lose weight. Nothing had helped me.

I certainly didn't want to join a group. I had heard about the ones where they pin little pig buttons on you if you haven't lost weight that week. I certainly didn't want that. And I didn't want to go to a group where they told me everything to eat or not to eat. I'd had enough humiliation. I didn't want to have to wear a pig button or be reminded that I had failed.

Well, *Free To Be Thin* was not what I expected. They told me the program was supposed to be a tool to help rebuild me so I could follow God. They told me I wouldn't be following a program as much as I would learn to follow God and hear what He was saying to me personally.

Through *Free To Be Thin* I learned to hear from God. I was taught to ask God how much I should weigh instead of trying to figure it out myself. I also learned how to ask God what to eat. I was amazed. I *can* hear from God!

In one year with *Free To Be Thin* I have lost 100 pounds. People tell me I'm not the same person at all. My personality has changed. I've learned what commitment means and I've learned diligence.

As an added bonus, my wife Toni has lost 60 pounds. We have been brought closer together because we are in the Word together every day. We've learned more about each other and the Lord than ever before.

Losing 100 pounds changed this man's life. He now feels free to be all he can be in Christ, released from the prison of fat and too much food.

Here's another story that is all too familiar. A woman testifies:

I have always been overweight. I was married at the age of 19 and became ill shortly after that. Being in bed without any activity I gained 50 pounds. Along with the 50 pounds came the feeling that nobody loved me, including my husband. I became jealous, lazy, nagging and very hard to live with. I tried to diet when my health returned but without any success.

My life was so miserable I didn't care what I looked like. I wore dirty clothes, kept a dirty house and didn't care about my home at all. When I became pregnant I gained another 50 pounds. I was able to lose 47 pounds after the birth of my daughter, but when I became pregnant with my son I gained 40 pounds. It seems as though I have been on diets all my life. I think I tried every diet I ever heard of.

One day in 1980 I met a girlfriend whom I had gone to school with. She had lost weight and began to tell me about a weight-loss group that she attended: *Free To Be*

Thin. From the first meeting I felt more love and support than I had ever felt before when I tried to lose weight. My life slowly began to change. I learned how to cry out for God's help. Because of my new attitudes, the Lord healed my marriage and delivered me from jealousy. I began to care about myself and my home.

Today I am 91 pounds lighter, and all because I learned the principles taught through the Overeaters Victorious ministry. I believe God has given me a new start.

Sometimes when you're tempted to quit or to say "I can't," or "It's too hard to stay on this eating program," remember what the Lord already has done. The Word of God says you can do all things through Christ who strengthens you. Sometimes you say you can't do all things—and in your own strength, you can't. But the Word of God insists you *can* do all things *through* Christ.

In order to develop diligence you need to fill your mind with the Word of God. It is essential for you to stretch your faith daily, and faith comes by hearing, and hearing by the Word of God. You are called to diligence. God is faithful to His Word. He can be trusted.

You're Under Construction

In the book of Ezra we read how the temple in Jerusalem was rebuilt. This temple was made and built by human hands. You, however, are a temple formed by God himself:

- "*. . . the temple of God is holy, and that is what you are*" (1 Cor. 3:17).
- "*. . . for we are the temple of the living God; just as God said. 'AND I WILL DWELL IN THEM AND WALK AMONG THEM. . .'*" (2 Cor. 6:16).
- "*Do you not know that you are a temple of God, and that the Spirit of God dwells in you?*" (1 Cor. 3:16).

Why does losing weight parallel the rebuilding of the

Temple at Jerusalem? Because God is rebuilding you.
You're His special project.

Notice the people God chose to rebuild the temple. They
were the Jews Nebuchadnezzar had taken to Babylon as
slaves seventy years earlier. God said they'd return
(2 Chron. 36:20–21) and they did. Most of these Jews had
been born in and lived in bondage all their lives.

King Cyrus of Persia, the man called to officiate the
rebuilding of the temple, sent out a proclamation to everyone asking for his valuables as freewill offerings for the
rebuilding project. The Jews, who were eager to restore
the house of God, responded overwhelmingly with their
silver, gold, goods and cattle.

You may have to give up something you value when
you decide to build your temple God's way. You may have
to say good-bye to those restaurant dinners at which you
eat everything from soup to mints and then waddle, stuffed
and groaning, to the car. You may have to give the Lord
your expensive taste in fine chocolate, your *gourmand-
esque* knowledge of French patisserie, your treasured recipes for southern pecan pie and apple fritters.

Everything changed for these temple workers. The first
things they did after accepting the task of rebuilding the
temple was relocate. They had to change their lives in
order to accommodate the work at hand. Their lifestyles
changed: their work, play, choices, time schedules, loca-
tion and habits.

When your temple is under construction, you'll experience changes, too. Major changes will include: (1) controlled shopping habits; (2) regular meal times; (3) no more
impulsive snacking; and (4) no more eating in restaurants
where the food is unhealthy and dripping with calories.

You will encounter emotional changes as well as di-
etary changes, changes of your mind, heart and soul. God
wants a *complete* reconstruction job. Change includes diligence. No temple was ever built without diligence.

What Is Diligence?

The dictionary defines diligence as being constant in effort to accomplish something. It is attentiveness and persistence. It is perseverance. Diligence is an "active" noun. It is something you understand only while you are *doing* it.

Toni had prayed, "Oh, please, Lord, let me have the diligence to sit down and just read the Bible." She had not enjoyed daily Bible study before, although she had been a regular churchgoer. Studying the Word on a daily basis and praying was not a habit. She needed to rebuild her temple but didn't know how. Now Toni daily reads the Word, writes in her journal, and has experienced a life-change she never knew possible. She is wearing a size 7/8, though she was certain she'd be a 16/18 forever. She enthuses, "I never knew that I could have a personal relationship with Jesus. I never realized that He could help me get a whole new body."

Toni's husband Jeff weighed 330 pounds and wore a size 52 before joining OV. In 11 months he lost 126 pounds. Toni has lost 60. Jeff says:

> I had to change. I had always eaten anything that was in front of me. The pattern we had established for our life was to eat . . . anything we wanted at any time. It was just our natural way of life. We ate constantly.

Diligence is preparing yourself for the times when you may not want to stay on your program or keep your commitments to the Lord. Toni and Jeff had lost their little boy in an accident and the couple ate incessantly after the child's death. Jeff recalls, "People brought over cakes and pies, cookies and casseroles and we ate everything. For two weeks people offered their condolences and we ate them." Toni began smoking again and eating more than ever before.

Jeff says:

I really began to see how personal the Lord is when we started attending the *Free To Be Thin* group. The program is so individual. The Lord showed us how to eat, because He is an individual God. I love the Lord so much for that. He treats us like we are special.

Now Toni and Jeff have another son and are living a new life full of joy and love. "We were diligent to stay on the program," says Jeff, "and I learned that diligence is not a bad word."

Give Yourself Permission to Change

Read the first chapter of Genesis and consider the changes God enacted in one week. He changed emptiness into life. In your journal record the changes you want to see in your life, for your habits will change as well as your weight. For instance, if you are tempted to overindulge when in a pizza restaurant, you will change your habits and no longer go to a pizza restaurant.

Lynette had lost 50 pounds but was down only to a size 22½. She had been diligent in losing her first 50 pounds, but says:

I still felt like a blimp. I just can't think of myself as thin unless I really work at my attitudes. I have fat days— such as a skinny morning and a fat afternoon. It's not that I eat, it's that I *feel*. Some days I feel fatter than I really am.

As part of your temple reconstruction program, analyze your attitudes. Worthwhile change will depend on your attitudes. Mary explains:

I have always associated fat with negative. When I experienced something negative I automatically registered it in my mind that it was because I was fat. Any unkind word or unhappy experience I associated with the fact that I was fat. So when I say I'm feeling fat it means that I'm feeling unhappy. It means I'm feeling rejected and I'm feeling frustrated. Usually if I feel fat I will be feeling angry or depressed, too. So often being fat makes me think that life only begins when I'm thin.

Change is certain to take place when you give your eating habits to God, because He calls you to a life of freedom.

It was for freedom that Christ set us free; therefore keep standing firm and do not be subject again to a yoke of slavery.—Galatians 5:1

Change your way of thinking to think of yourself as a free person.

When the Jews received orders to rebuild the temple, the first thing they did was "rise up" (Ezra 1:5). They faced the challenge—they did something. You also get out of bed to face the day, get out of your chair to do your projects, get into your car to go to work. In other words, you rise up and do something. Diligence exists where there is *doing*. Where bondage was a way of life for you, where eating meant defeat and disappointment to you, you can now rise up to meet this new challenge to rebuild your own temple. Bondage may have been a way of life for you, but you can change.

You have responded, just as the children of Israel responded when God spoke to them. You have said yes, and are rising up to begin work. You are going to be under construction. Possibly you have already lost weight, or are just beginning to lose weight. Or maybe you aren't sure you're ready to change your eating habits. Allow God to speak to you—through His Word, this book, through *Free To Be Thin* and the Overeaters Victorious program.

In your journal, write the word *change*. Then answer the question, Am I ready for change? Do I resist change? What in my life and habits will distract my temple rebuilding project? What might interrupt my commitment and hinder diligence?

One OV'er's journal says, "Even when I have not stuck with the teachings I have learned in the Word of God, the teachings have stuck with me." Another woman's journal says, "Even when my behavior has not been in line with the Word of God, I can say I'm sorry. I am learning to really believe God's Word. I find myself choosing His way more frequently in spite of myself."

The testimonies of men and women on the OV program reveal the deep work God does in His people. Even though God has much yet to do in each of them, there is much He has already accomplished. You also can experience victory because of Jesus who gives overcoming ability. Success and diligence go hand-in-hand. You can change. In yourself you are powerless to initiate a reconciliation with God, so yield to Him. Your body belongs to Him.

> *However, the Most High does not dwell in houses made by human hands (Acts 17:24). As the prophet says: "Heaven is My throne, and the earth is My footstool. Where then is a house you could build for Me? And where is a place that I may rest? For My hand made all these things."*—Isaiah 66:1–2a

When you are tempted to resist the Lord, it is probably because you have not been diligent to study and understand what God is telling you about yourself. Ask yourself:

• When am I usually tempted to resist God?
• Do I resist counting calories?
• Do I resist being diligent in my Daily Power Time?

The Apostle Paul exhorts, "I urge you therefore, brethren, by the mercies of God, to present your bodies a living and holy sacrifice, acceptable to God, which is your spiritual service of worship" (Rom. 12:1). Sacrifice is an *act* which follows a decision. Diligence is that act. When you submit yourself to God, you surrender to Him. Can you surrender yourself to diligence?

The Altar of Your New Temple

An altar is a place of sacrifice, cleansing and worship. It is also a place where commitments, decisions, are made.

You have an altar in your life where you make decisions, where you worship the things most important to you. In the book of Ezra we read the altar was the first thing the Israelites built. They knew the altar, the place of worship, was the heart of the temple.

In Ezra 3:3, it tells of the people worshiping God morning and evening. Worship is a daily experience. Your worship time is your Daily Power Time. From the very beginning of OV, the Daily Power Time has been a priority. In this chapter of Ezra, the altar is placed on a foundation. Even if your foundation is in ruin, you must have your Daily Power Time altar experience.

You Have All the Help You Need

In Ezra 3:7–11 it is clear that the people were not without help. Neither are you without help. Just as the Israelites hired carpenters and masons, you are not alone in your weight-loss endeavor. In a time of weakness you may feel you are without self-control, but that is the time you need to turn to the help God has given you. You can be diligent. You can walk worthy in the manner of the Lord in your eating because you have help. As the Israelites had help in rebuilding the temple, you have help in rebuilding your own temple with God.

1. *You have the finest materials.* The Jews brought cedar from Lebanon. *Your* cedar from Lebanon is the food you eat. It should be of select quality as the wood used in the temple. The finest, very finest cedar, is yours as you choose the most wholesome foods for your body. Natural foods, vitamin and mineral supplements (if necessary) and your new awareness of what you are eating will prove to be your most treasured materials. Some OV'ers bake their own bread. Others grow their own vegetables. If you don't have garden space, start window gardens. Some OV'ers grow their own sprouts for added nutrition in their diet;

others grow fresh herbs and vegetables on their patios and window ledges. The materials God has for you are the best because your temple deserves the best.

2. *You have overseers of the work.* Like the rebuilders in the book of Ezra you need a supervisor for the project. God has given people to help you: teachers, pastors, counselors, friends, or OV partners help insure your temple is rebuilt properly. Such people will encourage you when you feel discouraged and help you when you feel you can't help yourself.

God always works through people. It is not His will that you journey alone toward freedom. The Holy Spirit works not only within you but through the people around you. He wants your temple rebuilt and He has given you helpers to make sure the job gets done. Don't neglect seeking the wise and comforting words of your pastor and friends who understand your commitment to serving God in your eating habits. Don't turn to someone who is insensitive. Don't turn to someone who has no understanding of or experience in temple-building. You would not appoint a child who has never built anything as the supervisor of a construction project. Include those who want to see you reach your goals. Mature Christian friends will help you reach them.

3. *You have God's guidance.* You will daily experience insights through God's Word. The foundation you are building on is the Word of God. You are laying your foundation when you choose to build through His Word. A change will occur within you as you obey God in your eating habits, because you have set your mind on God's ways. The Holy Spirit is building you as you change your attitudes and make your will one with His. Your lifestyle will change forever.

Pray: "Father, in the name of Jesus, how may I please you today? I choose to be diligent in my eating commitment because I know you are concerned with the smallest details of my life. I give myself wholly to you now, Lord, to learn more about diligence and pleasing you in all areas of my life, so my temple will reflect your glory. Amen."

nine

Strength to Face Discouragement

The Opposition

Now the altar has been set up—the first step in rebuilding the temple and reestablishing a nation. Everything appears to be on schedule. The appropriate materials have arrived, the experienced supervisors are on the job, and the fear and worship of the Lord is established. Suddenly the mongrel Samaritans arrive on the scene. Accepting their offering of help would mean compromising with idolaters. This may be one of the most crucial points of your *Free To Be Thin* program. What kind of opposition will you encounter?

In Ezra 4:2, the opposition comes in the guise of helpfulness. Have you ever been tempted to lose weight any way you can, as long as you lose it? Neva went so far as to have intestinal bypass surgery. She suffered horribly as a result. After years of agony she finally found the solution in Jesus Christ. Diligence has made the difference for her, and it will for you. Being ready for the battle, for the opposition, fortifies you when you are tempted to turn to other kinds of help for your weight problem.

As you recall previous times you tried to lose weight, remember how discouraged you became. You slipped and fell, yielded to temptation, binged, confided in the wrong counselor, avoided proper nutrition or exercise, and turned to methods that haven't blessed you. The programs you have attempted have been the wrong ones.

A brochure on my desk tells me a certain powdered drink is the answer the overweight world has been waiting for. However, this material does not tell us the statistics of deaths and serious health problems that have resulted because of the radical nature of the program.

Magical, quick weight-loss plans are never from God. They do not include Him. God has given us abundance and the devil always wants to take it away. The devil wants to starve you and God wants to feed you. You are not learning how to diet on the *Free To Be Thin* program; you are learning how to eat, possibly for the first time in your life. You are learning that eating is a blessing and not a curse.

While on your *Free To Be Thin* program, we ask you not to use any other types of weight-loss methods. Supplement your food plan with moderate doses of vitamins and minerals, but unless your doctor prescribes a particular diet, please do not use any other program. The Lord Jesus is the director of your eating plan, and if you deviate from the *Free To Be Thin* program, you will find yourself losing weight, but gaining it back. There are many methods for fast weight loss. If you become deceived by their promises, you will bear the fruit of them. An empty promise produces an empty result.

You will learn you are not counting calories in order to be victorious, because you already are victorious. You will learn you are not choosing to be diligent in your Daily Power Time in order to conquer, but because you already are a conquerer.

The opposition's words in Ezra 4:2 are, "Let us help you" (NIV). How subtle. Ezra 4:4 says, "Then the peoples around them set out to discourage the people of Judah and make them afraid to go on building" (NIV). Discouragement can be a blinding experience. The blind cannot lead the blind.

Have you ever heard these discouraging words?

"Watch out or you'll lose too much weight and get sick."

"You're taking this *Free To Be Thin* too seriously."

"You'll be sorry if you lose all that weight and get skinny, because maybe your husband (or wife) won't like you anymore."

"You might fall into sin if you get thin and gorgeous."

"Look at how you are robbing your children. They don't get to eat cookies or bake cakes anymore."

"How come you won't eat more? I prepared this food just for you!"

"Are you going to let your diet stand between us and our friendship?"

The most deadly opposition of all is the statement, "You shouldn't try to lose weight because you were meant to be fat."

Ezra tells us there were counselors hired specifically for the job of discouraging the workers. They worked hard to thwart the rebuilding of the temple. You know which people discourage you. Not only do you face opposition in your program, you may have to encounter accusations as the workers on the temple in Ezra 4:6 did: "You just want to be thin so you can be better looking." Or, "You just want to lose weight so you can feel superior to people who haven't lost weight" (In other words: "You're guilty of pride.")

Ezra 4:23 tells us the Israelites were forced to stop their work. The work on the house of God in Jerusalem came to a dead halt until the second year of the reign of Darius king of Persia. What compels you to stop?

You are your primary and most vicious enemy. Stop blaming your "slump" on your husband who said, "You never bake for me anymore." You can still bake for your husband, but keep your mind set on diligence. If your spouse or friends say, "Let's go out to dinner," respond with a suggestion to eat at a place with a good salad bar. Circumstances, embarrassing situations, and boredom have proven to be deadly opposition for the person intent on weight loss. But believe your temple will be rebuilt because you are doing it with the power of the Holy Spirit.

Even though the work on the temple in Jerusalem was delayed, it was not delayed forever. "Let the temple . . . be rebuilt!" said the king in Ezra 6. The story has a happy ending. The Jews rebuilt the temple and prospered under the leadership of Haggai.

Haggai was a great leader and a godly man. It is essential that you listen to the preaching of a genuine servant of God. It may mean you'll have to change churches. It may mean you'll have to leave a comfortable situation you have enjoyed for many years. You need the power of the Holy Spirit in your life, for your own strength is not enough for you. The strength of your leaders is not enough for you if change is not taking place in your life. You are responsible to find that servant of God under whom you can be a student. It is not enough to go to church; you must be associated with a church that preaches the complete gospel of Christ according to the Word of God.

The Completion of the Temple

Joy and celebration describe the completion of the temple. The people were so excited at its completion that they celebrated and praised God with all their hearts. They offered magnificent gifts at the dedication. They appointed priests and rejoiced in the holiness of the temple. The sons of Israel returned from exile and joined those who had built the temple to worship the Lord God of Israel. They had their passover together and it was an unmatched holy day.

Wherever you are right now in your *Free To Be Thin*

program, God is giving you the diligence to complete the building of your temple. *You* are the temple of God. "For it is God who is at work in you, both to will and to work for His good pleasure" (Phil. 2:13).

Whenever evil comes in like a flood, God raises up a standard against it on your behalf. Remember, the opposition against you will end when you face it and expose it for what it is. With the power of the Word of God, expose the opposition you are facing. You know the Word of God because every day in your Daily Power Time you are studying the Word and praying. You are being persistent in *doing*. That is diligence. You are rebuilding. It may take time, but you are going to do it. You'll rejoice as these women do:

> I reached my goal weight five and a half months after I started my *Free To Be Thin* program. I lost 58 pounds. The first week I lost 13 pounds, and I was so shocked I nearly fell off the scale. For the first time in my life I started understanding what food meant to me. The calories and journal and Word of God all put together helped me to rebuild my mind as well as my body. I've got a brand new temple!

Those words were from a grandmother with four children and three grandchildren. She tells how her weight had been up and down all her life. She shared how she had lost weight in the past by skipping meals and starving herself.

Jean agrees:

> I'm five foot ten inches and when I began my *Free To Be Thin* program I weighed 207 pounds. I could never wear pants because I was pear-shaped. Now my temple is no longer pear-shaped [and] because Jesus has fulfilled His promise in my life, I am free to be thin and free to allow my testimony to shine through me. My mother joined *Free To Be Thin* too and not only did she go from 212 to 160, she was able to come off the blood pressure and thy-

roid pills she had taken for so long.

Carolyn confides:

> I discovered it was very easy to eat one slice of bread instead of a whole loaf. I discovered that I could go to the supermarket and not eat the groceries on the way home in the car. I discovered I did not have to eat before I went to bed and I did not have to eat my main meals between my main meals. My temple is new inside and out.

God sees your temple as already finished. He is already rejoicing and celebrating. Lift up your head because the Lord is celebrating your accomplishments. When He says you are an overcomer, you are. He is at this very moment bringing you from where you are to where He sees you finishing. When God says He is completing a work in you (Phil. 1:6), He is!

> **Don't put off living
> until you're thin.**

If your temple is under construction, enjoy yourself. Don't put off being attractive until you have lost more weight. Your temple is being rebuilt and every building block you are building with is beautiful. You do not have to wait until the day the temple is finished to appreciate yourself. It's not true that when you're thin your life will be more valuable, that when you're thin everything will be great. The truth is, everything is the same when you're thin as when you're fat unless the Lord Jesus has done the rebuilding from the inside out. If you are telling yourself you are going to buy yourself something new to wear once you lose weight, go buy it now. And don't buy it in the size you will wear when you are thin; buy it in the size you are now. You will feel good about yourself now. Buy good clothes from underwear to outerwear.

If you are really a size 18, don't continue to wear your size 22½ clothes. Buy something new. And when you out-thin those, buy some more, when possible. Be generous with yourself within the responsible limits of your budget. Your temple should be a place of joy and beauty at every stage of construction. If you've got 10 pounds or 100 pounds to lose, be beautiful right now.

You Are a Blessing

A pastor's wife said she had constantly encountered situations in which people would insist, "Have a little bit of this," or "I want you to try my (rich sauce, chocolate cake, cobbler, etc.)" or "How did you like the dessert I made?" or "Won't you just have a taste of this?" or "Here, have some more. You can always diet tomorrow."

She told how she had to regularly reaffirm her commitment to the Lord. She realized that without diligence she would be a chubby victim of opposition and fattening recipes forever. She knew her temple was being threatened. She says:

> But now that I have reached my goal weight I am amazed
> at the difference in my attitudes. My temple is safe and
> on a firm foundation. I have changed and become more
> in control and more assertive; I have a better rapport
> with people. I have discovered it's a blessing to say no,
> and I really don't offend anyone. I like myself and people
> like me, too.

Believe now that defeat is ended for you. This pastor's wife discovered being strong wouldn't offend anyone. Her new temple was a blessing, not a curse. God is at work continuing the labor on your temple. He is squashing the opposition.

Praise the Lord your temple is being rebuilt. You're under reconstruction. He is doing everything in His power to help you realize what He has already given you. Ezra 8:22 says, "The good hand of our God is on everyone who looks to him" (NIV). The good hand of God is on you right now as you rebuild your temple while looking to Jesus.

Pray: "Father, in the name of Jesus, I thank you that I can overcome all opposition because you say I can. I thank you that I can rise above the cares of this world and actually stay on my *Free To Be Thin* program, even though it seems hard. Thank you, Lord Jesus, that you are pouring out your Spirit upon me and you care about me. Thank you for King Cyrus, so many years ago, who was used by you to prophesy the rebuilding of the temple. Thank you, Lord, that I am a temple-builder and that you want to be my supervisor. Thank you for wanting to rebuild and make new in me that which has been in shambles. Thank you, Lord, for celebrating my victory even before I am a perfected temple. In Jesus' name, amen."

ten

The Problem of Patience

Free To Be Thin—Again

Maybe you have felt as the woman who wrote this letter:

> . . . I wish I could talk to you face to face. I wish I had somebody who could understand this "thorn in my massive flesh." I started my *Free To Be Thin* program and have really fallen flat on my face. It has been awful, horrible and everything else terrible. The first three weeks of Bible study and being obedient in what I ate were so good. I felt better than I had ever felt before. The Lord gave me so much strength—it was truly wonderful, and I thank you for your ministry that is so desperately needed in my life.
>
> But when things were going so well for me, something happened in my life that made me feel really rejected. So what did I do? I turned to food instead of Jesus. In two days I ate almost everything in sight. It's so hard to confess this. I had planned on writing up a fake calorie account sheet and fasting so I could lose what I'd gained, but I knew I could not do that.
>
> I don't understand why I do things like this. The hard part is forgiving myself—and admitting that I really am addicted to food and only the Lord can help me. Please pray for me. Sometimes I just don't know what to do.

If you have never been tempted to overeat while striving to obey the Lord and lose weight, you're not like the rest of us. The woman who wrote the above letter wrote out of her agony because the weight she had worked so hard to lose, she had now regained. The last words of her letter are, "Today I am starting over again."

For this woman, there is no tragic ending. Her story can be a success story. Luke 1:37 says, "Nothing will be impossible with God." What do you do when you feel you are a hopeless failure? What do you do when you feel you can't make it? First Corinthians 10:13 tells us:

> *No temptation has overtaken you but such as is common to man; and God is faithful, who will not allow you to be tempted beyond what you are able, but with the temptation will provide a way of escape also, that you may be able to endure it.*

There really is hope no matter how much you ate yesterday or this morning. "Common to man" means there is no temptation you face that somebody else doesn't face too. You are not alone. Re-read chapter fifteen, "What to Do When You Blow It" in the book, *Free To Be Thin*. We are in this together and even right now as you are reading this book, you have a brother or a sister who is struggling with the same temptations you are.

In 1 Corinthians 10, Paul summarizes the story of the Israelites following Moses to the Promised Land. They "all ate the same spiritual food and all drank the same spiritual drink" (1 Cor. 10:3, 4a). They were baptized into Moses in the cloud and in the sea, and the spiritual rock which followed them and from which they drank was Christ himself. Now doesn't that sound to you like an ideal situation? How much more spiritual could someone get?

They were living in one of the most amazing, and glorious moves of God in the history of mankind. They were "of one accord" ("common"), yet we read that "with most of them God was not well-pleased; for they were laid low in the wilderness" (2 Cor. 10:5). They grumbled, committed immorality, tested the Lord, worshiped idols and craved evil things.

But how is that possible? Why would they be so ungrateful when God was blessing them so wonderfully? Because a blessing is always something interpreted by the "blessee." The Israelites didn't consider themselves blessed. They didn't know the good and the beauty which could be theirs if they would only trust the Lord wholly. The Bible says, "Now these things happened to them as an example, and they were written for our instruction. . ." (1 Cor. 10:11). We can say we understand the Israelites' rebellion because we've done the same thing. We've lied on our calorie account sheet, or eaten four bowls of cereal and six pieces of peanut butter toast *after* dinner. We've known what it's like to be tempted and to rebel. Does that mean there's no hope for us? Is God angry? Has He given up on us?

Is God Angry with Us?

You and I were not created for defeat. Numbers 14:29 describes the Lord's disappointment that His people had chosen the wilderness instead of Him. But God did not erase their names from His book, for *"the Lord is long-suffering and slow to anger, and abundant in mercy and lovingkindness, forgiving iniquities and transgression. . ."* (Num. 14:18, Amp.).

The Israelites floundered and fell in the wilderness, and made the worst of it. The Lord who loves to be gracious and merciful wanted to forgive them, but they chose to remain in their predicament. When you find yourself laid low in the wilderness, tell the Lord, "I am in the wilderness, but you said you are faithful and will provide a way of escape for me. I will not remain in the wilderness." Here are some helps. Repeat them aloud:

1. I will immediately ask the Lord's forgiveness when

I become "laid low" in the wilderness.

2. I will seek new understanding through the Word of God. I will look for new incentives and fresh guidance in my Daily Power Time.

3. I will forsake all rebellion. I will not be afraid to admit when I detect rebellion in me. I will act immediately and not remain in my sin.

4. I will immediately apply the new principles I'm learning regarding my eating habits. I will daily apply what I learn and not postpone until tomorrow.

5. I will remember God is patient.

6. I will not be overtaken by temptations to overeat.

When Are You "Overtaken"?

"No temptation has overtaken you. . . ." Overeaters know what it's like to be overtaken. One lady writes:

I am 100 pounds overweight, and have tried everything to lose. As soon as I lose weight I gain it back. It's terrible to be fat. Even worse than being fat is the guilt I live with knowing I misuse my body that God gave me.

We have read hundreds of letters of guilt-ridden men and women overtaken by the temptation to eat too much. We receive countless letters from men and women all over the country crying for help.

You're not going to be totally overtaken, thrown into the pits of the wilderness, unless you willfully decide that's where you want to stay. We've never met an overeater who wanted to stay in the pit. Most people want to get out but need a way. Jesus is that way. Sometimes you might think that God asks the impossible of you. He asks to be Lord of your eating habits. You reply, "You ask too much, Lord." But is it too much?

"Nothing will be impossible with God" (Luke 1:37). Tell yourself now, "Nothing is impossible with God. All things therefore are impossible for me without Him."

You may be telling yourself that getting those last 15 pounds off is an impossible task. It's beyond what you are able to do. It's a mountain too high to climb, a job too laborious and unpleasant to attempt.

When Neva founded Overeaters Victorious, she had no idea of the vastness of the project ahead of her. What began with three women in her living room grew into a worldwide ministry. She could have been tempted to tell the Lord, "I'm not able to do this." She may have thought, "This is an impossible task to help thousands of people lose weight. It's okay to work with a few, but how could I possibly help people all over the world?" God has been faithful.

Temptation is common to us all, and one of the most common temptations is to tell ourselves a task is impossible. Nonetheless, in spite of that temptation to think something is impossible, *God is faithful, and He will make a way of escape.*

We received this encouraging letter from a woman in Louisiana:

> I know you get plenty of letters like this but I have read *Free To Be Thin* by Marie Chapian, and I know now that God will help me in my desperate battle against weight. I didn't think I could take off the 20 extra pounds I have on my body but now I know I can. I am a Christian and I have prayed every day about my weight problem. Somehow I could never get victory over it. Now I know the Lord will help me. I am going to listen to Him and *I am going to do it!*

Another woman from Washington, D.C., writes:

> . . . I have been on diet pills and for the past three years they have been affecting my health. I have tried to get off the pills, but I feel psychologically bound to them. In spite of these I have steadily gained weight and now am 35 pounds overweight and addicted to diet pills. Is there any help for me?

A man in California writes:

> I am a pastor and my battle with weight has been a fif-
> teen-year one. I have at least 90 pounds to lose. I thank
> you for a biblical perspective on my sin and a practical
> solution. *I know I'll make it. . . .*

With the Holy Spirit guiding and helping you, you have
all the power you need to handle temptation. There is
nothing beyond Him. Jesus forgives you when you ask
Him, and He also does not tempt you beyond what you are
able to handle. When Jesus was in the wilderness, He did
not stay there. He fasted 40 days and 40 nights and turned
it into a long prayer meeting. Afterward when the devil
tempted Him, He was not tempted beyond what He was
able. It is interesting to note that after fasting 40 days
and 40 nights, the first temptation Jesus faced involved
food. In the Garden of Eden, Adam and Eve were tempted
to doubt God's Word and eat what God told them not to
eat. Jesus, unlike Adam and Eve, did not go for the food,
but for the Word. The Word was His escape from temptation.

Satan will line up temptations for you like dominos in
a row. If you believe the first one, over it topples onto the
second one which topples upon the third one and down
they go until there are no dominos standing and you are
not only fatter, but more miserable than ever and filled
with disgust. The first temptation the devil topples on your
thinking is similar to his ploy against Eve: "Did God say
you couldn't eat that?"

Some Common Temptations

The first area the enemy strikes is your thinking. Listen to these tempting thoughts:

"Why don't you just go ahead and eat that yummy stuff
even though it's fattening? After all you're *hungry*."

"Go ahead and binge. Tomorrow you can fast."

"Eat now. Record on your calorie sheet later." (Free To

Be Thinners avoid this trap by *planning* what to eat.)

"Ice cream is much more soothing to your stomach than fruit or vegetables."

"Salads just aren't satisfying."

"You can't help your big appetite. It's just something you were born with."

"So what if you deviate just this once? It won't hurt you."

"You'll never lose weight. Fat just runs in your family."

"Did God really say you couldn't eat that?"

The Escape

First Corinthians 10:13 promises God will provide a way of escape. You may be tempted but you have a faithful God who has the escape hatch wide open for you. God gives you the help you need in the most intense time of your trial—when you follow your appetite only. You're in trouble when the temptation is the biggest thing in your life. When food is your every thought it's time to find that escape hatch. Read these words aloud:

> *You will seek me and find Me, when you search for Me with all your heart. And I will be found by you.*—Jeremiah 29:13–14

Call on Jesus! Reread the first chapter of this book. Your Daily Power Time is essential. Don't waste one second before you call on the Lord for help. When you are tempted to overeat, use this verse we've paraphrased and personalized as fortification:

> *I do not let sin rule as king in my body to make me yield to its cravings. I am not subject to its lust or evil passions. I do not offer or yield my body members to overeating but offer and yield myself to God. I have been raised from deadly habits to perpetual life. I present my body and its members to God as instruments of righteousness.*
>
> —Romans 6:12–13, authors' paraphrase

Your escape from sin is the Word of God. Satan tries to convince you before you fall into your wilderness of overeating that it really doesn't matter at all if you fall. He will try to convince you overeating won't hurt a thing. Here is another fortification at those times:

> *I am persuaded that neither life, nor death, nor angels, nor principalities, nor things impending, nor binges, nor guilt, nor self-condemnation, nor failures, nor Hershey bars, nor cookies, nor Coca-Cola, nor banana cream pie, nor Christmas, nor Thanksgiving, nor birthdays nor pot-luck suppers, nor anything else in all creation will be able to separate me from the love of God which is in Christ Jesus.*—Romans 8:38–39, authors' paraphrase

Just as Jesus answered Satan's lies with the Word of God, so can you.

When you overeat, binge, gorge yourselves, you are guilty of sin. Gluttony is sin. The truth is, you would be a perpetual wilderness dweller were it not for the truth that Jesus forgives your sins for the asking. He died for your eating that chocolate cake down to the last crumb. He hung on the cross for that pain you feel after eating until you can hardly walk.

God does not always work environmentally, rearranging the world around you in your favor so you will not be tempted to overeat. Instead, He works from the inside, making you strong and capable to meet temptation head-on and defeat it. You may be tempted to pray, "Lord, why don't you take this appetite away from me?" Instead, you can say to yourself, "I am not exempt from temptation, but I have the power within me by the Holy Spirit to be above it, to stand against sin."

You *will* win over your struggle with food because God is faithful. "If we are faithless, He remains faithful" (2 Tim. 2:13).

If you focus your attention on your shortcomings and the times you've yielded to temptation, you'll feel bad.

You'll feel guilty. You may even feel condemned. But God is faithful. He fortifies you. He cleanses you. He disciplines you and teaches you a new way of life because He is faithful and loves you more than you will ever know.

Wanda is acquainted with the mercy of God. She writes in a letter:

> I went on my first diet when I was 20. I was 13 pounds overweight. Three months later I was 18 pounds overweight. *That's how I really became fat, by going on diets.* Each time I lost weight, I gained it all back plus five extra pounds.
>
> I went on Weight Watchers about ten years ago and lost 55 of the 65 pounds I wanted to lose. I gained most of it back. I heard about *Free To Be Thin* through a friend who lost 40 pounds on the program. Before I started I gained five pounds. I figured, I might as well eat now because I wouldn't be able to eat later.

Wanda is thrilled today because after six months she lost 40 pounds. After a year she writes:

> God in His mercy started a whole new life for me through *Free To Be Thin.* When my husband and I go to dinner, I am satisfied with 410 calories. I have so many victories I can't name them all. I have been a Christian for 25 years, but I have never been able to lose weight and keep it off. The Lord is wonderful because He had patience with me when I was so rebellious. He understood when I was trapped in my fat eating habits. He had mercy. . . .

Wanda felt she didn't deserve mercy. She didn't feel she deserved to be thin. God is a loving and forgiving God, and He does not turn His back on you when you need Him.

Pray: "Thank you, Lord, for being faithful and patient. Thank you for teaching me to be disciplined and to hear your voice in times of temptation. Thank you, Lord, for the tempting times so I can overcome and taste victory. Help me turn temptation into a growing experience, Lord, to produce a deep, lasting work in my heart and mind. This is the time when I am really learning what you mean by patience. Thank you, Father, for what you are teaching me. In Jesus' name, amen."

eleven

Learning to Eat, Not Diet

Free To Be Thinners do not diet, they learn how to eat. We have never yet met an overweight person who didn't know how to diet. Most overeaters have tried dozens of diets and are aware of the futility and discouragement of dieting.

Elaine made an important self-discovery as she read over her journal of the last year. She had already lost 50 pounds and still didn't feel she was a success because she had 25 pounds to lose. But as she reread her journal, she realized the years of being fat had not hurt her nearly as much as dieting had, that she had hurt her health as well as her emotional state of being by constantly dieting.

Her lifelong obsession had been to lose weight. It was difficult to allow herself the freedom not to diet on her *Free To Be Thin* program. She had been attempting diets since the age of 14 and had set some patterns that were emotionally rooted.

"I started hating my body when I was about 13 years old," she says. "I was only slightly overweight then, but I became very self-conscious when a boy in my class jokingly called me fat. I was just crushed."

Elaine was not obese at the time, but started thinking

of herself as fat. She later became obese.

You may have learned to hate yourself when very young, developing a distorted picture of yourself at a time when outward appearance was so important. The teen years are self-conscious years, and you may have remained, emotionally, a teenager too long. You are free at any age, though, to see yourself through the compassionate eyes of Jesus.

The Problem with Dieting

A serious consequence of too much dieting is that the dieter places a moral value on food. She becomes "good" when she sticks to her diet, but "bad" when she doesn't. The dieter becomes obsessed with food, and normal responses to the appetite for food become distorted. The degree of that distortion varies in each person, but many people do not know what it is like not to be dieting, believing if they aren't doing something about their weight, they're "bad." To be "good," therefore, is to diet.

The misunderstanding is that one must be in a state of penance in order to be good. Dieting becomes a form of punishment, just as being fat is. Since fat is bad, one is bad if fat. Bad people get punished; hence, perpetual dieting.

But here is good news! You are free to be thin when you are free to love yourself, even if overweight.

Elaine told a group of women:

> I can now talk nicely to myself and say loving things instead of always telling myself what a rotten person I am. I used to ask myself, "How could I be such a fat slob?" I always said to myself, "How could I let myself get so ugly? Who will ever love me when I'm so fat?" Now I say things like, "I'll make it. I can obey the Lord. The Lord is with me. I can stop punishing myself. I'm really more than free to be thin."

Another serious consequence of dieting is the destruction of the body's natural balance. Chronic dieters are often chronically obese and run the risk of developing diabetes, high blood pressure, hypertension, and heart disease. Strokes are also linked to obesity, and research indicates the incidence of gall stones is six times more likely to occur among the obese than among people of normal weight.

Because a dieter is more interested in thin than in health, she often neglects sound nutrition, thereby robbing her body of health, energy and vitality. The health hazards are many (physical, mental, emotional), and the person who perpetually diets is usually the one with low self-image. Jesus specializes in low self-images and that is why when you decide to become free to be thin, you throw away your old diets and diet mentality.

It took Elaine a year to realize she was truly free to be thin, because losing weight permanently is a process, not a single act. Dieting focuses on a single act, but lifelong weight loss is accomplished one day at a time, and she can maintain her new thin self one day at a time.

You can be in harmony with your body and enjoy yourself as you lose weight God's way. Dieting has not made you thin in the past and will not make you thin now. Dieting is frustrating and unsuccessful if you gain what you've lost after you go off your diet.

Jesus has a solution for the problem of dieting. He also offers us a new definition for the word success. You can experience success in a new way every day. The Lord wants you to live a life of success and contentment. He wants you to feel good about yourself.

In the past you may have considered thin to be success. Some people will say, "I'm not a successful person because I can't keep my weight down." Another equally false statement at the opposite end of the spectrum is, "God isn't interested in what I eat. He doesn't really care if I'm fat or not."

God cares about every area of your life. When you are

truthful with the Lord, you need not be ashamed to face yourself and your inadequacies. You can tell the Lord you are sorry when you have been unruly and disobedient in your eating. If you confess your sins, He forgives and cleanses you from all unrighteousness (1 John 1:9). Being honest with God will help you to go forward, knowing He is a loving God, willing to forgive. He is eager to comfort, strengthen and encourage you. Christ paid the price for you to conquer your food obsession.

What Is "Failure" Doing in Your Vocabulary?

Let's get a new interpretation of the word failure. Instead of viewing failure as total defeat, why not see it as a challenge to change? You may think because you're prone to eat too much that you are a failure as a person.

God doesn't fail. He offers a way to be successful even when you think you are a total failure. God's power and ability is bigger than your eating problem. Sometimes you wait too long before you turn your problem over to God. You are so accustomed to thinking of yourself as a failure that you naturally assume it's your permanent condition. The Lord wants to encourage you with words of truth and success. He is eager to save you from every affliction you can name, including overeating.

For Thou dost save an afflicted people. But haughty eyes Thou dost abase.—Psalm 18:27

When you are overweight you are not as healthy or energetic as you can be. What weight is healthiest for you? At the beginning of the *Free To Be Thin* program you learned that the first step to becoming weight-loss was to hear from God how much He wants you to weigh. It is God who sets your goal weight, not you alone. In that way, success is His. You then learn to ask the Lord what you should eat. You learn that in order to fulfill God's perfect plan for your life, it is necessary to obey Him in every aspect of your being. For too long your fatness held you in rebellion and you grieved, hurt, and suffered insecurity and pain. Fat can be an affliction.

Success at Last

But there is hope for the afflicted! There is blessing for the afflicted. God saves you out of affliction. This promise is yours. He is right now working to save you from every fat lie you've ever believed, from every fat action, behavior and thought. He is showing you principles from His Word that lead you to happy and successful choices. He is revealing himself to you every day during your Daily Power Time. His guidance and love save you from the affliction that has entrapped you.

Whether you have 10 pounds or 200 pounds to lose, the Lord is leading you. He who has begun a good work in you will never quit! Even if you get tired or tempted to give up, or become convinced your goal will never be reached, God will not give up. He is still saving you from your affliction.

Success is the Lord's. Study and memorize these verses!

I am poor and needy; yet the Lord thinketh upon me: thou art my help and my deliverer.—Psalm 40:17, KJV

God is our refuge and strength, a very present help in trouble.—Psalm 46:1

He will regard the prayer of the destitute, and not despise their prayer.—Psalm 102:17, KJV

And all things, whatsoever you shall ask in prayer, believing, ye shall receive.—Matthew 21:22

The Lord Jesus gives you every opportunity to succeed. As your refuge and strength, He will never allow your afflictions to overtake you when you call to Him for help. Success is realizing that food does not possess you. You were created to be possessed by the Holy Spirit. You were created for success, and success is a choice.

God's Humbling Methods

Psalm 18:27 tells us God saves an afflicted people, "but haughty eyes thou dost abase." Haughty means having or showing great pride in oneself. It means having contempt for other people. You are being haughty when you consider yourself and your problems more important than others and their problems. Haughtiness is arrogance, self-centeredness.

The Scriptures say God isn't pleased with this condition and He will humble you if necessary. When this happens you might feel as if the rug had been pulled out from beneath you. God's method of humbling is to give you a good look at yourself. He removes all your pretensions and shows you the real thing. When you begin eating foods you shouldn't, and snacking when you know you shouldn't, God steps in with a holy "ahem . . ." to get your attention. Your pride doesn't frighten Him. He will bring it out in the open so you can deal with it.

Pride is a Christian's enemy, but your protection is the Word of God. Psalm 40:1–3 tells us the way to avoid pride is to keep close to God. And to do that you must recognize your need, your pit of helplessness, even as the psalmist did:

I waited patiently for the Lord;
And He inclined to me, and heard my cry.
He brought me up out of the pit of destruction,
Out of the miry clay;
And He set my feet upon a rock
Making my footsteps firm.
And He put a new song in my mouth,
A song of praise to our God;
Many will see and fear,
And will trust in the Lord.

God is hearing your cry, bringing you out of a pit of destruction, setting your feet where your feet ought to be, and giving you a new life. His humbling methods are intended for you to come to grips with your need for the Lord. He wants you to see Him for who He is. It is then that you can align yourself with His ways instead of your own.

Give thanks to the Lord, for He is good; for His loving-kindness is everlasting.—Psalm 107:1

God's humbling methods are to give you the happiness and the joy He wants you to know as a child of God. His humbling methods teach you to thank Him in all things. Thank Him for every ounce of fat you lose, and thank Him for the marvelous fact that you have finally set your mind on listening to and obeying Him in your eating habits.

The Brightness of Success

"For Thou dost light my lamp" (Ps. 18:28) is a promise God is giving you because His light is wisdom and knowledge. Think of the emotional darkness in which you once lived when you had no way out of overeating. One OV'er explains it this way:

When I first started watching my weight, I read all the books and listened to all the experts tell me how to do it. One expert would tell me never eat white flour or sugar and another would tell me it wouldn't hurt me. One expert would say don't eat artificial sweeteners and another would tell me to drink diet sodas and use artificial sweeteners. One expert would tell me to eat nothing but protein and another would say don't eat protein only. The the Cambridge Plan came out and I was told this was the answer I had been waiting for. Later I was told to beware because it wasn't good for my health.

I didn't know what to do. I prayed to the Lord and said, "Lord, where do I find truth in all this?" Now I realize that it is God who illumines me, shows me the way and teaches me. I have an inner knowledge now I didn't have before. God has opened my eyes to what's right and good. I'm out of that confused state.

Another OV'er says:

I had no idea how to eat the right way when I was fat. I had so many addictions to food that I had lost my good sense about eating properly. Some days I would eat six or seven candy bars for lunch and not even realize I was starving my body. I ate until I was full and it didn't matter what I ate. Then I'd fast and eat nothing at all for a couple of days. Yes, I was *afflicted*. I desperately needed wisdom and illumination.

Your Safety

Thy Word I have treasured in my heart that I may not sin against Thee.—Psalm 119:11

God's Word is the wisdom you hunger for. If you will treasure the words of God in your heart, you will not sin against Him or yourself. When you hide His Word in your innermost being, your thoughts will more readily respond to His leading. His silent urgings will become familiar to you. You will know Him and what He is telling you.

I have inclined my heart to perform Thy statutes forever, even to the end.—Psalm 119:112

Your attitude changes when you hide God's Word in your heart. His Word is your safety and your protection. In this safety, your attitude changes toward God, yourself and food. You will find your attitude changing toward the people around you, as well. With the Word of God planted in your heart, you will find you can understand your own behavior better. You will see how you have used food as a reward and a comfort. You will see how food has provided companionship. When you incline your heart to perform the statutes of God, you will see that eating has been a major interference of contentment and peace in your life.

Have you been eating out of anxiety, bitterness or

worry? The Word of God reveals that you are not to be anxious. You are not to worry. If you are bitter or unforgiving, you can ask God, "What am I unforgiving about? My overeating behavior shows me there is something amiss." God will show you and you will live according to His laws, to "perform His statutes forever, even to the end."

Performing His statutes *to the end* means not just until you reach your goal weight, but *forever*. You are most safe when living in the statutes of God with His Word hidden in your heart. It is your place of protection and joy. It is your place of lifetime success.

Pray: "Dear Lord, infill me with your Holy Spirit to enable me to keep your Word and to love your statutes. You have saved me from the affliction of being fat, and I choose to walk in my place of victory and success. You have heard my cry and you promised to bring me out of the pit of destruction. I will trust you and obey you and choose your success methods for every area of my life. Thank you for giving me strength and for saving me from myself. In Jesus' name, amen."

twelve

The Starvation Trap: Bulimia and Anorexia

Free to Be Fatter

Cindy was a beautiful 18-year-old from an upper middle-class family in California. She was in her first year of college and earning good grades. She had high standards and goals and was considered by everyone who knew her a "clean, wholesome girl, well-liked and friendly." Her parents considered her a model child, but noticed she was getting thinner than she had ever been in her life. When she came home at school break, her personality had changed. She sulked and pouted and seemed restless most of the time.

Cindy didn't return to school after the semester break. To the horror of her parents, her condition, known as anorexia nervosa, had gone too far. She was hospitalized four days after she arrived home. Her friends at school had known she had an eating disorder, but didn't know how serious it was. They could hardly believe it when the hospital called and informed the stunned family that Cindy's heart had given out and she was dead.

People write letters to OV frantically begging help for the insidious disorders of anorexia and bulimia. They are both serious conditions and can cause permanent damage, even death.

Anorexia nervosa is a syndrome of self-starvation. It is the abnormal rejection of food. Bulimarexia, or bulimia, is a combination of names coined from the Greek meaning ox hunger or insatiable appetite. The bulimic gorges on food, sometimes eating thousands of calories at a time and then vomits before digestion takes place. Self-induced starvation, anorexia nervosa, is often followed by such binging and purging behavior.

These eating syndromes are becoming widespread in the United States, especially among young women in high school and college. Bulimia is not a new syndrome, for the Romans practiced gorging and vomiting during their banquet orgies. Anorexia nervosa is not new either, and was first described as an eating disorder in 1870.

The anorexic or bulimic person has exaggerated fears of becoming fat, even though she is close to normal weight. A high percentage of people with these eating disorders are women. They overreact to society's dictates of beauty and femininity and feel exaggerated pressures to be thin. They are often addiction-prone to drugs or alcohol; they have impulse problems and usually come from families where eating, alcoholic or emotional problems exist.

In a study made at UCLA of 800 bulimics, nearly every woman interviewed said her eating disorder started in her teen years as a result of a preoccupation with dieting. The social pressures of being thin were overwhelming her. One out of five of the bulimics became unable to control the urge to vomit, thus becoming addicted to vomiting, a compulsive behavior like alcoholism and drug addiction. The addiction to gorging and vomiting is harder to control than alcoholism or drugs because one must eat to survive, and to the bulimic, eating is inseparable from gorging.

The Causes of Eating Disorders

The central issue behind an eating disorder is not food. The person and her family may spend most of their time worrying about, discussing, nagging and arguing about food and body weight, but food is not the central issue. Self-starvation and binge-purge behaviors are directly related to an intense desire to be special, to unrealistically high expectations of achievement.

Most physicians and mental health workers who specialize in eating disorders agree that issues underlying anorexia and bulimia include poor self-esteem; feelings of helplessness; and the struggle to win power, approval, admiration and respect from family, friends, and society. Eating is the method the anorexic or bulimic chooses to gain these goals.

Trying to solve serious problems through bizarre food behaviors is typical of the bulimic or anorexic. Instead of using mature coping strategies, she typically falls into distorted thinking and behaviors, including compulsive vigorous exercise.

One ex-bulimic writes:

My eating behaviors anesthetized my feelings. One way I kept myself going when I was exhausted, weak and hungry was by thinking about and visualizing food I could eat later on. No one ever knew I was hungry and hurting inside; no one ever saw how hopeless I felt when there was nothing on my "safe" list, so I knew I had to endure the light-headedness and emptiness even longer. No one knew as I exercised frantically, I was so weak that I had to force myself to do it. I didn't tell anyone because I knew they would try to make me stop . . . or eat . . . so I lied to them and I lied to myself. I told myself to ignore the pain. I could no longer tell the truth from a lie. I adamantly believed bread would make me fat. (After all, most diets tell you to cut it out!) So I told myself bread was bad and I told my friends I did not like bread. I came to believe it. (I would only eat breads on binges and then feel guilty because I knew bread equals bad equals fat.) Now I eat an average of four slices per day and I'm not fat. Something was wrong with my thinking then. Yet, somehow, by exchanging the truth for lies, I was able to continue to anesthetize the pain. Almost all of my thoughts were on food, exercise, weight and/or binging. My communication with people was mostly superficial and it became unnatural for me to discuss my feelings.[1]

Is There Hope for the Anorexic and the Bulimic?

Unlike compulsive eaters, the anorexic expresses her preoccupation with food by self-starvation. The behavior is characterized by a fear of food as well as an obsessive interest in food. Like the compulsive eater, many anorexics engage in all-out eating binges. The shame and self-disgust causes her to fast, vomit or take laxatives.

The Apostle Paul wrote, "But I say, walk by the Spirit, and you will not carry out the desire of the flesh" (Gal. 5:16). There is a direct connection between walking in the Spirit and breaking a harmful habit. Bulimia and anorexia have been termed as addictions because of the lifestyle these syndromes engender. When struggling with addiction of any kind, the Bible tells us we can be addicted to the Holy Spirit and thus supplant the power sin had over us. God knows each one of us and He knows each of our needs. There is hope.

It is impossible for God to lie. [Therefore] we may have strong encouragement, we who have fled for refuge in laying hold of the hope set before us. This hope we have as an anchor of the soul, a hope both sure and steadfast.— Hebrews 6:18, 19

Call on Him

Answer me when I call, O God of my righteousness! Thou hast relieved me in my distress; be gracious to me and hear my prayer.—Psalm 4:1

---

[1] K. Kim Lampson, *The Hopeline Newsletter*, 1982.

Keep on Keeping On

*Forgetting what lies behind and reaching forward to what
lies ahead, I press on toward the goal for the prize of the
upward call of God in Christ Jesus.*—Philippians 3:13–
14

Think on a Higher Level

*And so, as those who have been chosen of God, holy and
beloved, put on a heart of compassion, kindness, humility,
gentleness and patience.*—Colossians 3:12

In the name of Jesus, who has the power to save us
from every evil, every disaster, every enemy, you can be
free from abnormal eating habits. Repeat these truths to
yourself every day:

I Have Deliverance:
"I command you in the name of Jesus to come out of her!"
And it came out at that very moment.—Acts 16:18

I Have Healing:
*"By the name of Jesus Christ the Nazarene, whom you
crucified, whom God raised from the dead—by this name
this man stands here before you in good health."*—Acts
4:10

I Have Salvation:
*"I am the door; if anyone enters through me, he shall be
saved, and shall go in and out, and find pasture."*—John
10:9

I Have Power to Overcome:
*And who is the one who overcomes the world, but he who
believes that Jesus is the Son of God?*—1 John 5:5

I Have a New Life:
*I have been crucified with Christ; and it is no longer I who
live, but Christ lives in me; and the life which I now live
in the flesh I live by faith in the Son of God, who loved me,
and delivered himself up for me.*—Galatians 2:20

Becoming a New Person with New Needs

The Bible says when you became a Christian and were filled with the Holy Spirit, you became a new creation. "Therefore if any man is in Christ, he is a new creature; the old things passed away; behold, new things have come" (2 Cor. 5:17). You are a new person and can "put on the new self, which in the likeness of God has been created in righteousness and holiness of the truth" (Eph. 4:24).

Your new self wants to be in control: *"Put on the new self who is being renewed to a true knowledge according to the image of the One who created him"* (Col. 3:2).

You have a new kind of hunger when your life is at the foot of the cross. *"Blessed are those who hunger and thirst for righteousness, for they shall be satisfied"* (Matt. 5:6).

The new person you have become in Christ also has new desires. *"One thing I have asked from the Lord, that I shall seek; that I may dwell in the house of the Lord all the days of my life, to behold the beauty of the Lord, and to meditate in His temple"* (Ps. 27:4).

There is no habit too big to defeat when the Holy Spirit is in control. Your needs are met in Christ because He promises you shall not be in want of any good thing (Ps. 34:10). The Lord knows your failures and your victories. His right hand will save you because He promises when you walk in the midst of trouble He will revive you (Ps. 138:7).

The Lord has searched you and known you. He knows you when you sit down and when you rise up. He understands your thoughts and is acquainted with all your ways (Ps. 139:1–4). Christians often are afraid God will not accept them because of their problems with carnality. This is the reason you need the Holy Spirit. His power is greater than your fears, your doubts and your carnality.

Free to Be Fatter and Happier

Help for the bulimic or anorexic requires understanding and knowledge of the problem, as well as a spiritual awareness of the fact that the devil and his cohorts are at the root of all sin. The sin against one's body may not appear to be as bad as sins such as murder and stealing, but God does not measure sin in value. He sees any sin as rebellion, period. The author of sin is the devil. If you allow yourself to be defeated constantly by the devil, you will find it increasingly difficult to hear the voice of God.

If you are a parent, family member or friend of a person suffering with anorexia nervosa or bulimia, realize nagging and cajoling will not help. You can help most by listening and caring, but you cannot expect to solve the problem by yourself. The person with the eating disorder needs sound, professional help.

If you are attempting to cope with anorexia or bulimia, Jesus stands at the gate of your heart, waiting to help you in every problem, whether it be fear or stress, or striving to achieve, or desire for acceptance, or worry—every sin and failure you have known. Write your thoughts in your journal and tell the Lord everything on your heart. Then write the truths God is impressing you with as you study the Scriptures included in this chapter. Write down the promises of God. Meditate on them.

Set some goals for yourself this month. Look at those goals every day. What do you want to begin afresh right now? What is your goal for every day of the month? Be sure to take time to rest, to pray, to talk to friends and to study and meditate on the Word of God.

Nancy wrote after her experience in the OV program, "My expectations when I first enrolled in this class were desires to be changed—to be rid of bulimia. To be free from the fear of getting fat if I gave up bulimia."

When Nancy was asked if her expectations were fulfilled she wrote, "Praise God! I stand in victory of no more vomiting, laxatives, or misuse of diuretics! As I am willing to receive His truth and obey His way, the weight and fear will disappear." Nancy received the strength and encouragement she needed from other group members. They prayed and helped her to realize how valuable she was to God and how important that she be free from satanic control. She is now free to be thin.

The Lord sustains all who fall and raises up all who are bowed down. The eyes of all look to Thee, and Thou dost give them their food in due time. Thou dost open Thy hand, and dost satisfy the desire of every living thing.
—Psalm 145:14–16

thirteen

Freedom Is "Normal"

Not the End of the Road

Gloria moans after getting on the scale and seeing she's only lost a half pound in seven days. "When will I ever be *finished* with this weight-losing business?" she asks herself. "I hate it! I starve myself, deny myself, go without, and I only lose a half pound. When will I ever be able to eat normally again?"

Remind yourself right now that your eating habits are a priority concern in your life. One of the mistakes you can make during your *Free To Be Thin* program, and after you've reached your goal weight, is to forget your goal. Keep your goal in mind during each day and remind yourself you are still in the *process* of altering your lifestyle. Veteran dieters such as Gloria know how to lose weight, but losing the weight is not the end of the road. Your lifestyle needs constant attention.

Gloria has to realize "normal," as she thinks of it, is unrealistic. She sees "normal" as being able to eat whatever she wants whenever she wants. With such thoughts, she will gain back what she lost once she reaches her goal weight.

For years you may have seen food as a comfort, and as

a problem-solver. Realize now you will never be finished with controlling your eating. There is never an end of the road where control is concerned. Don't look forward to a gluttonous family reunion between you and your favorite foods.

"Normal" is not being able to eat whatever you want, and it is not starving either. Gloria is good at starving, just as you may be. But keeping weight off is a lifestyle; starving is not. Most diets don't teach that thin is a lifestyle. The end of the diet is typically the end of the road.

The diets provide methods for peeling off pounds, but once you've reached a goal, the methods you used to get there don't offer any help. You can't live on boiled eggs and watermelon the rest of your life. Sooner or later you're bound to run into a peanut butter and jelly sandwich or an avocado dip or some other calorie-laden food. You'll have lost 20 pounds but you'll be hungry and if there is Christmas candy or a box of cookies on the shelf, watch out. It may take seven days to lose a half pound but only one unbridled afternoon to gain five. Remind yourself you are still on the road, still committed to obeying the Lord. This is not a dream or a wish. It is real.

Remind yourself every day:

For you were formerly darkness, but now you are light in the Lord; walk as children of light (for the fruit of the light consists in all goodness and righteousness and truth), trying to learn what is pleasing to the Lord. And do not participate in the unfruitful deeds of darkness, but instead even expose them.—Ephesians 5:8–11

On your *Free To Be Thin* program, losing weight may sometimes be an up-and-down process, but you will be equipped with the skills of picking yourself up, dusting yourself off, and starting anew several times before you reach your goal. Eventually you must learn new habits, *lifetime* habits. First John 1:9 is always your refuge, and when you see the need, start anew. Start refreshed, forgiven and ready to learn to please the Lord again.

Yes, You Can!

If you've bounced back-and-forth on various diets and are screaming, "I can't do it!", we assure you, "Yes, you can." God is there with His arms out, ready to take you from the darkness into the light. You can learn what pleases Him, and when you do, you learn what is real and you learn about yourself.

"Yourself" is a wonderful person, full of hope and good things, and a person who is in control (by the Holy Spirit's power). A thin, young woman named Betsy says:

> People ask me, now that I'm thinner do I feel like a different person? I have to tell them, that the truth of the matter is, I'm different because I'm now *real*. The fat person I was just wasn't the real me. The thin person who is in control now is the real me.

Another woman named Ella writes on her response sheet:

> When I was fat I thought size nine was utterly tiny. When I finally went from a size 22½ to a size nine, I realized you can be a size nine and still be fat in your mind. I have lost weight before and panicked I'd be fat again. Being thin didn't make me free. I couldn't trust myself to go off a diet. Once when I reached my goal weight after dieting for three months, I went out on a binge and gained ten pounds in two days. The real me was still fat.

You can be thin outside and fat on the inside. The best way to be is free—free to be thin. Wishing to be thin won't do it.

How Hungry Can You Get?

For many people, the reason to lose weight is the very same as the reason for their overweight. "I want what I want, *now!*" Overeating, overspending, oversleeping, overindulging, overtalking, over-anything represents a spiritual hunger the Lord wants to satisfy. Walking as "children of light," we become conscious of pleasing the Lord, and when that happens, we change. Our attitudes and appetites change.

Don't be too hard on yourself if this change takes time. One woman told us that when she awoke in the morning, she would scheme how to get something to eat before breakfast. She had been on her *Free To Be Thin* program one month and lost eight pounds. Now her mind was flooded with food fantasies. In the past she had awakened in the middle of the night to eat whatever she could grab from the refrigerator. Now she was sneaking calories by snacking between meals, at night and early in the morning. She had countless BLT's (bites, licks and tastes) which she didn't record on her calorie account sheet. She was not studying the Word or keeping her journal. She had missed her Daily Power Time for a week. She was heartsick to see she was gaining weight instead of losing, but she didn't realize that her hunger wasn't hunger at all, but a need to hear from the Lord.

How hungry are you? Are you hungry enough to admit your hunger is really spiritual hunger? Wishing does not have the power prayer does. You can wish you could lose 20 pounds, but eating 3,000 calories a day won't make your wishes come true. When you ask the Lord how many calories a day to eat, He will show you. He will also show you it is good to be hungry for God.

What Has Calories?

- BLT's (bites, licks and tastes) have calories.
- Food eaten while standing up has calories.
- Food eaten in the middle of the night has calories.
- Food eaten before breakfast has calories.
- Food "tasted" while cooking has calories.
- Food that isn't "filling" has calories.
- Food left on someone else's plate has calories.

- Beverages (except water) have calories.
- Food eaten and not recorded on the calorie account sheet still has calories.

A self-controlled person is not a person who lives continually in victory without ever stumbling. A self-controlled person is one who may stumble, but gets back up! Even if you are sneaking and snacking, eating food without counting calories, wishing instead of praying, and acting as though you're hopeless when you are not, the Lord is there to help you. He teaches you, because He knows you truly want to please Him and because He can turn your failures into victories when you allow Him to. Failure is not inevitable every time you open a refrigerator.

What is God's will for you *today*? Take time now to write the answer to this question in your journal. Instead of wishing you had control, longing to be a size five by New Year's, or lose 20 pounds by June, take action.

In the *Free To Be Thin* study, you were asked to make a Desire-Action worksheet. Repeat the assignment now. (See chap. nine, p. 70, in *Free To Be Thin*.) On one side of the paper write your desires. On the other side, write the action needed to fulfill each desire. Then write down what might stop you from attaining your desires. The "I wish" syndrome will stop you from attaining your goals. Turn your "I wish" list to "I will."

Here are some wishes you may reocognize:

I Wish . . .

. . . I were more disciplined in my prayer life.
. . . I had better control of my credit cards.
. . . I were thinner.
. . . I felt more attractive.
. . . I had a better job.
. . . I was a neater person.
. . . I had better attitudes.

. . . I had more control of my time.
. . . I had self-control in my eating.
. . . I were healthy.
. . . I got along better with _____.

Turning Wishes into Reality

Identify your dream. The Bible implies this:

Now to Him who is able to do exceeding abundantly beyond all that we ask or think, according to the power that works within us.—Ephesians 3:20

Don't be afraid to name what you are asking of God. He says He will do *more* than you ask.

Psalm 37:4 tells you to delight in the Lord because He will give you the desires of your heart. Acknowledge the desires of your heart and believe that what you ask of Him, He hears.

Psalm 44:21 tells you that God knows the secrets of your heart and Psalm 145:14 tells you He sustains and raises you up when you are bowed down. (Read Ps. 145:14–19.) Identify what you are longing for. God promises to fulfill your desires.

Sanctify your dream. When you know your desires are approved by God, you know you can live in confidence that He is hearing and answering. Pray and ask the Lord, as David did in Psalm 139, "Search me, O God, and know my heart; try me and know my anxious thoughts; and see if there be any hurtful way in me, and lead me in the everlasting way." God answers such a prayer. He will use people and circumstances to show when your desires are not right. David prayed, "Turn away my eyes from looking at vanity, and revive me in Thy ways" (Ps. 119:37). David constantly prayed that the Lord would keep Him clean in both thought and action. He wanted to be sure he was in the Lord's will. You can be sure, too, by praying in the same manner David did, "Search me, O God."

Meditate on the following verse:

Finally, brethren, whatever is true, whatever is honorable, whatever is right, whatever is pure, whatever is lovely, whatever is of good repute, if there is any excellence and if anything worthy of praise, let your mind dwell on these things.—Philippians 4:8

Confirm the dream. Turn your wishes into reality by experiencing the reality of God. When you confirm or ratify your dream, it is because you know, without a shadow of doubt, who God is. You know He is able to do all you ask of Him. When you seek Him, you find Him. When you fight against Him and His ways, you hinder the answers to your prayers, as well as the ability to live the lifestyle you desire.

One of the key concepts in a life-saving course is that a person fighting in the water is very difficult to save. The lifeguard is instructed to knock out the drowning person, if need be, in order to save his life.

Spiritually, you need to be rescued. Quit fighting and admit your need. Then your dream will be confirmed as you allow God to rescue you from disobedience, unbelief, failure, and every other negative weight. Proverbs 2:1–8 shows why God confirms your dream: He shields, guards, preserves, and protects every good thing in your life when you allow Him to.

C. S. Lewis wrote that when we accept heaven, we shall not be able to retain even the smallest and most intimate souvenirs of hell.[1] So dream a heavenly dream. Write down your dream. Let nothing rob you of the reality of your dream. No matter what you weigh now, God will make your dream of thinness and freedom a reality.

---

[1] C. S. Lewis, *The Great Divorce* (Macmillan Publishing Company, 1946).

fourteen

A Seven-Day F.A.D. Diet

A Fabulous F.A.D.[1] Plan That Is Actually Good for You

When you need a new start, a jolt of encouragement, here is a seven-day plan to help you. This special FAD plan is for you if you have (a) gained back some weight; (b) been on a plateau for a long time; (c) need to get started with a real boost; or (d) just need encouragement.

The rules for the FAD plan are:

1. Follow the Bible study closely.
2. Follow the daily instructions exactly.
3. Take liberal doses of your Spiritual Food Supplements many times a day (see Appendix).

The FAD plan is intended for seven days only, but it may be extended for one additional week. Two weeks is the longest time you should remain on the plan.

Day One

Bible Study: Isaiah 43:18–19
Instructions: Drink liquids only: tomato juice, apple juice,

---

[1]Faith Applied Daily.

lemon water, skim milk, bouillon, pineapple juice, grapefruit juice, or any natural fruit juice.

In your journal mark a special section for your FAD seven-day plan. On the pages record *daily* your thoughts and prayers. Record what God is showing you through your Bible study and what you are sharing with Him. Be sure to take massive doses of your Spiritual Food Supplements. Read them aloud and record them in your journal.

Day Two

Bible Study: Psalm 16:7–9

Instructions: Add to your liquid diet: nine ounces of lean meat or fish—broiled, baked or boiled. (Please, no lamb or pork.) Divide meat into two or more servings.

Record observations in your journal as you did in Day One. Remember, you cannot overdose on Spiritual Food Supplements.

Day Three

Bible Study: Psalm 22:23–26

Instructions: Add two large salads or steamed vegetables in any combination. Now your food plan includes liquids, two salads or vegetables, and two servings of lean meat.

Record your thoughts, prayers and inspiration from the Lord in your journal.

Day Four

Bible Study: Psalm 40:1–8

Instructions: Add breakfast: two ounces orange juice or other juice rich in vitamin C, one egg and one-half Holland rusk (toasting the rusk makes it taste better).

Continue your journal. The insights gained on this FAD plan should be enlightening.

Day Five

Bible Study: Psalm 28:7–9
Instructions: Add one piece of fresh fruit.

Remember, you are on this special plan to look to the Lord, not to the weight loss. On this day spend extra time with your Food Supplements and writing notes in your journal.

Day Six

Bible Study: Ezekiel 11:19–20
Instructions: Add second piece of fruit.

Continue, in your journal, writing out your prayers, thoughts, and what the Lord is showing through your Bible study. Remember your dream which God is turning into a reality.

Day Seven

Bible Study: Ezekiel 36:26–36
Instructions: Same as Day Six.

AFTERWORD:

After completing your seven-day FAD plan, answer these questions:
1. Did you follow the directions exactly?
2. What Scripture from your FAD Bible study meant the most to you, and why?
3. What other meaningful Scriptures helped you with this study?
4. Did you use your Spiritual Food Supplements?

5. What was the hardest part of the plan?
6. What was the easiest part of the plan?
7. Are you ready to advance to your next step of victory?

Here are some responses other OV'ers have written:

Martha:

Being able to eat without counting calories was not easy for me. It became easier through the Bible study because the Lord helped me to obey Him and not take this plan as a license to binge. I know God is the strength I need and He will help me.

Lois:

The Bible verses gave me strength to eat what I should. Psalm 40:1–8 is very special to me now. He has taken me from the bog and mire and put my feet on solid ground.

Donna:

The "Food Supplements" picked me up. The FAD plan was a little hard for me, but I lost weight and I feel better having eaten the right foods. I feel so much better about myself. I'm ready to go on to the next step of victory.

Dorothy:

Each day was exciting as I began to find God with new insight. I truly was not concerned about weight loss during the seven days because I was meditating on the Scriptures and really allowing the Lord to speak to me.

Marge:

I feel good! I lost six pounds. I enjoy my Daily Power Time with the Lord. I need prayer and strength, and this week especially helped me. My relationship with people has changed. I'm really excited about myself and I'm excited that God can help me start again.

Barb:

I have a choice, a godly choice that has been given to me. I am no longer bound by Satan's schemes to make me fat. I lost three pounds. Hebrews 10:36 helped me and I am so happy the Lord is enabling me to fulfill His will for my life.

Karen:

I am amazed at the changes taking place in my spirit already. I have been so aware all week that my body is being brought into subjection to my spirit. It has been so exciting to me. I am expecting great things to take place in my life spiritually. I knew if I made it through the second day I would have a major victory in my life. Praise God, I did.

Tanya:

I am so happy because this is the first time in my life I have ever fasted. It feels so good to know I can discipline myself and tell myself I can do without. All week long the Lord dealt with me about sweets. It feels so good to be free. I'm ready to go on to the next step of victory.

Lorene:

I feel real good because I made it without blowing it. The Lord talked to me about removing my old ways and walking in the new way. I am excited to go on from here.

Lynn:

I have lost six pounds and I'm overjoyed. What an encouragement and sense of victory promised in Ezekiel's words. God is my strength. It has been His work and His encouragement that have given me the jolt I needed. I know He will rebuild me and other people will praise Him because of His work in me.

Ann:

This week was not a total breeze, very difficult at times. I feel I am growing spiritually, sometimes slowly. Holland rusk is a real trial. Isaiah 43:18–19 stopped me from looking backward and gave me hope in the process the Lord has started.

Jerri:

I drank too much fruit juice and only lost one-half pound. I remembered while reading Ezekiel that my power comes from God's Spirit and not from me.

Your FAD plan can be a friend if you let it be. When you complete your seven days, call a friend and tell what God has shown you. Talk about your victories and blessings, not only to encourage yourself, but someone else.

Pray now and ask the Lord what new thing He wants you to do on your way to being free to be thin.

fifteen

Find a Partner

Pastor Ed Tedeschi said to a group assembled for a *Free To Be Thin* leadership conference, "Sometimes we get to the point where it is impossible to do any more alone. The encouragement of working together, the inspiration of sharing a task, the added energy, the strength that is shared may make the difference between the job getting done or not getting done. . . ."

Ecclesiastes 4:9 says:

> *Two are better than one because they have a good return for their labor. For if either of them falls, the one will lift up his companion.*

An OV group is really a gathering of partners. A group can simply be two or three persons meeting regularly at least once a week. The Lord doesn't expect anyone to be a loner. He wants His people to work together, to encourage one another because they need one another.

The Lord didn't just give the Bible and let you run alone. He said, "Forsake not the assembling of yourselves together." When you gather with others who desire to lose weight for the glory of God, you form a partnership.

We received a letter from a woman in Montana who said, "Please help me. I weigh 250 pounds and I'm desperate." We encouraged her to find a friend or relative who would be her partner on her *Free To Be Thin* program.

You need the support of another person to challenge you and keep you honest. You need another person to pray with you and help you fight the attacks of the devil.

Do not look for someone to be your parent. Your friend is your partner. The leader of a *Free To Be Thin* group shares only OV teaching and meets for mutual encouragement.

When a group becomes large, it is best to subdivide. Big does not necessarily mean success in *Free To Be Thin*. This program is geared for the individual, and each individual needs loving attention. The ideal group size is four to eight. One or two strong personalities can take over the meeting if the group gets too large and the timid souls will sit quietly in the background. A friend-partner won't let that happen.

Stick with the program. Don't give up. Encourage your partner to endure. One woman confided how easy it was for her to make friends. She told us people always liked her instantly and she had no problem getting along with new people. However, she had a problem *keeping* friends, and she wept as she explained how difficult it was for her to keep a long-term friend. "Once people get to know who I really am, they don't like me anymore." We advised her to be who she really is right from the beginning. Accept one another for better or worse, encourage one another to become all you can, including thin. You can do it because you are not alone. Your life always touches someone else's life.

A Promise to My Friend

You are my friend and I love you. When you are down I will help you get on your feet again. I will help you when you are weak. I promise to be consistent in my love for you. If you want to binge, don't ask me to be a part of it. I promise I will not be a partner to your failure, only to your success. I will not cook, prepare, buy or tempt you in any way with food that is not on your Free To Be Thin *program or in your best interest.*

I promise I will not be a stumbling block to you. I will daily pray for you. I am confident of the work God is doing in you, and I know He will continue it in you until you reach the perfect image of Jesus. I will keep a special place in my heart for you at all times.

If you should fail I will be there to help you and remind you of our forgiving Savior. When I am tempted to fail, I will remember my success is important to you. When I want to cheat or be negligent in my calorie counting, I will remember my diligence helps you to be diligent, too.

When you need me to be firm, I will be firm. I will always endeavor to be patient and gentle and compassionate. I will share with you the insights I receive through the Word of God. I will seek creative ways to build you up in the faith and encourage you. I always want to seek your good. Don't expect me to feed your self-pity (should there be any) and don't expect any fattening goodies from me. I will not feel sorry for you when you refuse a gooey treat that everyone else is eating. I will respect you and rejoice for you.

We will make it this time, my friend. We will make it because we are not alone. Jesus, you and I are friends.

sixteen

Maintaining What You've Lost

This chapter is specifically for the day you reach your goal or if you are now at your desired goal weight. It is designed to help you stay where you are and maintain what you have.

The Lord has rewarded me according to my righteous-
ness;
According to the cleanness of my hands He has recom-
pensed me.
For I have kept the ways of the Lord,
And have not wickedly departed from my God.
For all His ordinances were before me,
And I did not put away His statutes from me.
I was also blameless with Him,
And I kept myself from iniquity.
Therefore the Lord has recompensed me according to my
righteousness;
According to the cleanness of my hands in His eyes.
—Psalm 18:20–24

Where are your rewards? Because you have been honest and upright before the Lord, you have received the blessing of God. You have lost the weight you prayed to lose and you have reached your goal. You could not have done it without honesty toward God and yourself. You've been faithful with your calorie account sheet, faithful to

149

confess your shortcomings and failures, faithful in your commitment to Him and faithful in your Daily Power Time. The Lord has rewarded you because you have kept His ways. If you departed, you returned and now you're at your goal.

Your Reward

Galatians 6:7–9 presents the law of sowing and reaping. When you sow to the flesh (your old, selfish, carnal nature), you reap to the flesh. There are a number of ways to sow, including planting ideas in your mind. When you plant evil ideas in your mind, you will reap evil attitudes and actions. When you plant selfish, worldly ideas, you will reap selfish, worldly attitudes and actions. When you plant the Word of God, the thoughts of the Holy Spirit, in your mind, you will reap inner loveliness and power, as well as peace and love in your attitudes and actions. When God's Word is in your thoughts, in your innermost being, your habits will change, as well as your thoughts.

When you think about foods you shouldn't be eating, chances are you will eventually eat them. When you ask the Lord what foods you should eat, and you obey His instructions, you will succeed and receive a reward, both physical and spiritual. When you make your grocery list, invite the Lord to sit down with you so you can discuss with Him what you are going to buy at the store.

Pray about the people you are having over for dinner tonight. Should you really bake that fattening dessert for your company? If it isn't good for you, it probably isn't good for them, either. Your friends will live through an evening at your home without something fattening and gooey to eat. Let the Lord reward you and that reward will also touch the people you love.

If God tells you not to eat a certain food, it just might not be the right thing for others to eat, either. When the

Lord shows you which foods to eat and not eat, there usually never comes a day when you can ignore what He has shown you. God is making permanent changes in your eating habits. Your reward will be lasting, not temporary.

A *Free To Be Thin* group leader shared that when people come to her house they eat what she eats, because if it's good for her, she figures it's bound to be good for them. Even if her guests have no need to lose weight, eating the food God has specified for their hostess will not hurt them.

The Unholy BLT's

You may want to write in your journal today, "No BLT's!"

BLT, as we mentioned before, means bites, licks and tastes. One of the most important decisions you can make, now that you are free to be thin, is to stop tasting the food you cook. Do not eat while you cook. Do not eat while you shop. Do not finish junior's cheeseburger. Don't have a BLT before supper—or afterward. You may have to repeat this to yourself over and over because your old hungry self may loom up at the sweet smell of someone else's sandwich or chocolate bar. If you could see all the calories you have consumed unawares in bites, licks and tastes, you could probably feed three people for a year.

This Is Forever

Beth says:

I had been fat all my life. Up and down. About five years before I got married I lost 58 pounds and it took me over a year of starving myself. When I started *Free To Be Thin*, I had to eat three meals a day, which I was afraid of doing. I always thought I had to skip meals. I thought I had to starve. I can't believe how the Lord worked. Actually, I really can believe it because I am experiencing the reality of it. I lost the same amount of weight in only five and a half months and I have kept it off. I'm healthy now because I know and plan what goes into this body.

Tina tells us:

At last I am in control. I have found that being able to say no is a blessing and not a restriction. I don't say "Poor me" everytime someone else has dessert and I can't. It's more of a blessing that I can say no because I know I am obeying the Lord and He will reward me.

Ruth tells us:

I have a bona-fide love for Mexican food. It used to be that I could eat 3,000 calories at a sitting eating Mexican food. No more. When my husband and I go out for a Mexican dinner, I have a salad. I never knew I could eat the salad in my tostada only. I always felt obliged to eat everything in front of me, including the chips, the *guacamole*, the *quesadillas*, the potato skins and the beans. All this before the main meal! I am free now. I have reached my goal and I have stayed there. I discovered that I could be the total person I was meant to be in the Lord because He touched me through losing weight. The Lord used my overweight to get to me and I thank Him for it.

Helen declares:

I have maintained for three years. It really is a forever thing. When God does a work He doesn't do it just for a couple of weeks, a month or a year. It's forever. I really believe I will never be fat again. It took me a long time, but I finally *feel* thin. I will never be a compulsive sugar-holic again. I have learned to listen to the Lord and to experience what is pleasing to Him.

What Is Pleasing to the Lord?

Here are some tried-and-true tips for you as you continue to please the Lord in your eating habits. The Lord says you can understand what His will is: *"Do not be foolish, but understand what the will of the Lord is"* (Eph. 5:17). The Amplified Version of Ephesians 5:10 says, "And try to learn [in your experience] what is pleasing to the

Lord;—[Let your lives be constant] proofs of what is most acceptable to Him." When you are finally at the point of maintenance, it is vital that you know what the will of the Lord is for you. You already know what pleases Him; otherwise you would be listening to other people instead of the Lord. You would be pursuing other radical ways to lose weight fast or you would be smitten with fear that you will regain everything you have lost. Record in your journal the ways in which you have pleased the Lord.

How can you understand the will of the Lord, how to please Him? Romans 12:2 says to break your ties with this world and not to be conformed to it. You are to be transformed by the renewing of your mind, in order that you can prove God's will, which is good, acceptable and perfect. Here are some specifics on proving God's will when you have reached maintenance status:

1. *Eliminate empty foods, and empty calories.* Beware of filling foods that do not feed you. You can eat two dozen cookies and feel bloated, but four ounces of cottage cheese with some fruit will make you feel satisfied. Beware of the fattening "fillers."

2. *Try new recipes and foods.* One of the reasons you don't experiment with new recipes is old habits. You don't want to try anything new and daring. Nobody you know makes zucchini lasagna so you don't want to try it. (Be sure to use the *Free To Be Thin Cookbook* for some exciting new recipes, including zucchini lasagna.)

When God begins to change your eating habits, He will introduce you to new foods. Be open to new tastes and new recipes. There may even be certain simple foods you think you'll hate, yet those may be what God is giving you as a blessing. A counselor in the OV office hated cottage cheese for years. She didn't like the smell of it or want to be around anyone who was eating it.

One day at an OV leadership training seminar, she was served cottage cheese for lunch. She was so hungry she didn't know what to do. She prayed, "Lord, help me. I hate cottage cheese, but that's all I have here to eat." She suddenly realized she could eat cottage cheese, and has been eating it ever since.

There may be foods you have always detested, but now you may discover they are better than you thought. Be open to new foods. Try new recipes. One lady who tried the Copenhagen Cabbage Casserole in the *Free To Be Thin Cookbook* was delighted by its delicious taste. She said, "I thought I didn't like cabbage."

3. *Enjoy your new habits:* It usually takes 21 days to establish a new habit. If you have added more protein to your diet, give yourself 21 days to get used to it. If you are at your goal weight, give yourself 21 days at that weight to establish the habit of eating only enough to maintain your goal weight, and no more.

Once you have a set of new habits in operation, you can consider making new ones. When you have established a good breakfast, then you can concentrate on a good lunch. It is important that you take one step at a time, as well as one day at a time.

4. *Establish new habits without bragging.* It is difficult to be quiet when you are losing weight. (Reread chap. 21, "How to Talk About Losing Weight Without Being an Unbearable Bore" in *Free To Be Thin*.) When God does a work in your heart, it is best to be quiet about it until you are certain of what has taken place. When the work of God is solidified and you are experiencing a new heart and mind regarding food, then you can talk about it.

How to Know When You Have Reached Your Goal

You become a candidate for the maintenance phase of your *Free To Be Thin* program when you reach the physical and *spiritual* goals God has set for you. This is the time for you to establish all God has done in you. God wants to continue to move in your life and He wants to develop new spiritual awareness and beauty in you. You are now in total agreement with a lifetime eating plan. You no longer hate the idea of discipline.

You know you are ready for a maintenance program when:

- You no longer lie about the number of calories you're consuming.
- You habitually plan what you will eat for the day *before* the day begins.
- You do not feel sorry for yourself when other people are eating fattening things and you aren't.
- You don't miss your Daily Power Time.
- You are not threatened by your new thin self.
- Going to a restaurant doesn't ruin your eating plan.
- You have put fun into eating by being creative with your menu.
- You are eating healthy food and enjoying it.
- You fully realize weight loss is because of the Lord Jesus.
- You know what your danger signals are and are prepared for them.
- You are eating three meals a day.

Some Danger Signals

Be aware of those problems that caused you to overeat in the first place. Being on a maintenance program does not mean you throw away all caution and can now sit back and do nothing about your weight. Being on maintenance means you now understand yourself and your body, and you are able to "keep standing firm and . . . not be subject again to a yoke of slavery" (Gal. 5:1).

Some danger signals are:

Frustration. When things don't go your way and you are irritated, you may be tempted to take a quick trip to the supermarket. When plans go awry, and when you're not appreciated as you think you ought to be, you may become frustrated and hungry at the same time.

Boredom. When you are not interested in what you are doing, your mind may wander—directly to the kitchen. If you're not filled with purpose and motivation, you may become lethargic and succumb to temptation to overeat.

Self-pity. Beware when you are telling yourself, "Nobody loves me," or "I miss out on so many good things," or "Nobody cares if I'm fat or thin anyhow." (You can add your own self-pity sentences here that you know are danger signals to you.)

Overindulgence. When you tell yourself, "This food looks so good, I just can't resist," look out. Look out for the feeling that sweeps you away with the thought, *This tastes so good, I just have to have a little bit more.* When you overindulge, you are lying to yourself about the food and about what your body can handle.

Bitterness. When you are bitter and angry, and feel helpless about it, stay away from the goodies you once turned to for comfort. When you have been unjustly wronged, when your children don't obey, when the dog chews the heel of your new shoes, when the car won't start, when your best friends didn't invite you to a party they are having, realize you are setting yourself up for a binge. Avoid bitterness. Pray, "Lord Jesus, give me a heart of peace and contentment."

Hurt feelings. When you feel wounded, maligned, misunderstood, and your heart is broken, know that thoughts of food and eating may loom before you as a comfort. When the tears slide down your cheeks, know the refrigerator will seem like a friend. It's not.

Loneliness. When you are alone in your home and wish you had someone to talk with, be sure you don't choose food. When you are feeling left out or deserted, and sad about it, you are approaching a danger point.

Jesus is the author and perfecter of your faith. He doesn't expect you to have perfect faith without Him. When you are on maintenance, you do not have to pretend that everything is okay if it isn't. You can admit your danger signals and do something about them because you know there is a way of escape.

No longer must you smile and tell people everything is fine while hiding your true feelings. In counseling overweight people, an OV leader might ask, "How are things with you in general?" An obese person may answer, "Everything is great." The question then is, "If everything is great, why are you obese?"

Put this question on your refrigerator: *"If you're overeating, what's eating you?"*

Things in your life are not right if you are rushing to the kitchen instead of Jesus. This shows you are experiencing conflict, even though you are on maintenance. God isn't finished with you yet; He is still perfecting you. He is constantly teaching, changing and maturing you. You may want to have your own way, do things your way, ignore all you have learned from Him, but He is faithful and is perfecting you.

Here are principles of discipline to sustain you when you begin your maintenance program. Allow them to become your good friends.

1. Place yourself daily in God's hands.
2. Ask the Lord about the foods you can eat each day.
3. Feed daily on the Word of God in your Daily Power Time.
4. Pray without ceasing; communicate with God.
5. Don't be afraid to obey the Lord.
6. Resist the devil with all the spiritual weapons available to you.
7. Don't underestimate your danger signals—be ready to act.
8. Refuse self-condemnation.

9. When tempted, remember it is only temporary. Call a friend or prayer partner.

10. Tell yourself every day, *less is more.*

God wants to transform every detail of your life. If your weight is the only area of your life in which you sense He is working, you are not as free as you could be.

The Last Stronghold

"Strive to live in peace with everybody, and pursue that consecration and holiness without which no one will [ever] see the Lord" (Heb. 12:14). Your relationship with the Lord changes and blesses you, and also touches the lives of those around you. Your spiritual triumphs must affect your relationships with others as well as your relationship with the Lord. To live with peace is a great gift, but to give peace to those around you and to handle problems in your relationships through the Holy Spirit's wisdom and ability is like heaven on earth. Not only are you successful in preparing menus and eating plans ahead of time, not only do you pray before you buy groceries, not only do you buy wholesome foods and avoid binges, but you "strive to live in peace with everybody."

One *Free To Be Thin* woman happily writes on her response sheet:

> I lost 52 pounds and am at last at my goal weight. I just can't believe how loving my weight loss has made me. I used to be a bitter and resentful person and I didn't even know it. I feel at peace with myself and at peace with people. Thank you, Jesus.

Consider the relationships in your life that need to be touched by the love of God. Lay aside your old, selfish self. Don't be tempted to sit around and wait for God to strip you of old bitter feelings. Lay those feelings aside, just as Paul wrote in Ephesians 4:22: "Strip yourselves of your former nature—put off and discard your old unrenewed self. . . ." The real you, the self you are free to be, is loving, forgiving, content, and at peace.

Pray: "Thank you, Lord, that through the power of your Holy Spirit, I finally can maintain what you have given me. I can walk with a clear mind being renewed by the Holy Spirit daily. Thank you, Lord Jesus, that I am important to you and that the love and health you have given to me will touch the lives of other people, as well as my own. Thank you there is no area of my life with which you are not concerned. In Jesus' name, amen."

seventeen

Pressing On

Final Helps

Do you have a personal statement of faith? When you look at your life, do you see a list of do's and don'ts? A statement of faith is something you live, just like a do's and don'ts list. Your goals are something you live also. Your life unfolds after your goals are chosen. When you are free to be thin, you really can stay there. Here are some helps from Neva's list. Read them and add your own if you like:

- I look ahead at what I'm becoming and I refuse to look at the past and my mistakes. I strive daily to see how God sees me.
- I refuse to settle for anything less than God's goal for me.
- I refuse to fret or be anxious about anything. The Lord tells me I am not to be anxious about anything, but with prayer and supplication to make my requests known to Him.
- I maintain a thankful heart. Instead of self-pity, I spend time praising and thanking the Lord for all He is and is doing for me.
- I refuse a martyr-attitude. No sacrifice I can make

compares to the one Jesus made. The only thing I really give up is my own selfishness.

- I fix my mind on the positive. I do it on purpose because ordinarily I may not always see the bright side. I remain positive by allowing the Word of God to renew my mind.
- I take time to rest both physically and spiritually. I plan regular "mental health days." I do not want to become discouraged.
- I do not listen to people who generate doubt. I surround myself with people who are positive and uplifting. These people like to surround themselves with people who are positive and uplifting, too.
- I refuse destruction in any form in my life. I realize I need deliverance from old habits and I want always to be open to deliverance and help.
- I do not allow myself to experience spiritual hunger. If I take care of my spirit first, my spirit takes care of the rest of me. I plan for my Daily Power Time because I accomplish what I plan to do.
- I tell myself it's okay to be hungry. I will not be afraid to eat less and leave the table a little bit hungry.
- I refuse to be impatient, because God is doing a work in me that will last for all eternity. I refuse to allow the limits of time and space to make me impatient with God's work in me.
- I refuse to "do it my way." That's how I got fat, I did it my way. The more self-sufficient I was, the fatter I became.
- I will always put God ahead of my business. He is first in all things in my life. Having a thin body is not first, God is. Actually, we need to heed our bodies less and God more.

More Than Free To Be Thin

When you enter a restaurant in a strange town, nobody will know about your commitment to God and *Free To Be*

Thin. You could eat every pastry in the display case and who would care? But when you are free to be thin, you are free in all circumstances. You are *strong* and free. You are more than a conqueror. You have a higher calling.

The High Calling

If God has called you to be truly like Jesus, He will draw you into a life of crucifixion and humility, and put on you demands of obedience that sometimes will not allow you to follow other Christians. In many ways He will seem to let other good people do things He will not let you do.

Other Christians, and even ministers, who seem very religious and useful may push themselves, pull strings, and work schemes to carry out their plans, but you cannot do these things. And if you attempt them, you will meet with such failure and rebuke from the Lord as to make you sorely penitent.

Others can brag about themselves, about their work, about their success, about their writings, but the Holy Spirit will not allow you to do any such thing; and if you begin bragging, He will lead you into some deep mortification that will make you despise yourself and all your good works.

Others will be allowed to succeed in making great sums of money, or having a legacy left to them, or in having luxuries, but God may only supply you daily, because He wants you to have something far better than gold—a helpless dependence on Him— that He may have the privilege of providing your needs daily out of the unseen treasury.

The Lord may let others be honored and keep you hidden away in obscurity, because He wants to produce some choice, fragrant fruit for His coming glory, which can only be produced in the shade.

God will let others be great, but keep you small. He will let others do a work for Him, and get the credit for it, but He will make you work and toil without knowing how much you are doing. And then to make your work still more precious, He will let others get the credit for the work which you have done, and this will make your reward ten times greater when Jesus comes.

The Holy Spirit will put a strict watch on you, with jealous love, and rebuke you for little words and feelings or for wasted time, which other Christians never seem distressed over.

So make up your mind that God is an infinite Sovereign who has a right to do as He pleases with His own, and needs not explain to you a thousand things which may puzzle your reason in His dealings with you.

God will take you at your word; and if you absolutely sell yourself to be His slave, He will wrap you up in a jealous love, and let other people say and do many things you cannot do or say.

Settle it forever, that you are to deal directly with the Holy Spirit, and that He is to have the privilege of tying your tongue, or chaining your hand, or closing your eyes in ways that others are not disciplined.

Now, when you are so possessed with the living God that you are, in your secret heart, pleased and delighted over this peculiar, personal, private, jealous guardianship and management of the Holy Spirit over your life, you will have found the vestibule of heaven.

—Unknown

A Note from Neva:

A lady from a central California coastal town writes that she came to a *Free To Be Thin* class out of curiosity. Wanting to lose some weight, she was very intrigued with the concept that Jesus could be involved with her on such a personal level—that He really cared about helping her reach her goal. Some of the spiritual principles shared during the class session caused her to start thinking about the bondage in her life to smoking. She confided in her group leader who encouraged her to use those same principles in this area of her life. She not only lost the extra pounds, but she was able to quit smoking as well. And she wasn't just an ordinary smoker—she was smoking marijuana.

There IS more to being thin than just being thin! This dear woman—along with thousands of others (including me!)—has been learning about freedom from habits and bondages, being disciplined, hearing God's voice, living victoriously. She has also been learning about ministering hope and help to others. She is now leading a small group ministry within the Overeaters Victorious class where she first studied *Free To Be Thin*.

How about you? Are you ready to learn about the free, disciplined life? Are you willing to learn about recognizing others' needs and reaching out with help and hope? Are you ready to learn that there's more to being thin than being thin? Many have learned this and have been totally changed by the power of God. They are now free to be all that God wants them to be. You can too!

Neva Coyle

Spiritual Food Supplements

These "supplements" are to help you as you reach and maintain your goals. There's more to being thin than being thin.

My old unrenewed self was nailed to the cross with Jesus. My body which is the instrument of sin has been made ineffective and inactive for evil. I am no longer the slave of my fleshly appetites. I have died with Christ, and I also live with Him.—Romans 6:6

I do not eat for reward.
I do not need such rewards.
I have my reward!
I have holiness and eternal life.—Romans 6:22

I surrender and yield my appetite as an instrument of obedience to the Lord. I do not surrender to the demands of the flesh. I choose to be obedient to the Word of God. I crucify the flesh. I do not yield to the passions of the flesh. The flesh is dead.—Romans 7:6

I do not let sin rule as king in my body to make me yield to its cravings. I am not subject to its lusts and evil passions. I do not offer or yield my bodily members to overeating but offer and yield myself to God. I have been raised from deathly habits to perpetual life. I present my body and its members to God as implements of righteousness.—Romans 6:16

I do not surrender to temptations of the flesh, for I am not, nor will I become, a slave to the flesh. Rather, I choose to obey God. I choose the way of righteous obedience. Here I am, Father, what would you have me do?—Romans 6:16

I am a debtor, but not to the flesh. I am not obligated to my carnal nature—to live a life ruled by the dictates of the flesh. Because if I live by the dictates of the flesh I will surely die. But if by the power of the Holy Spirit I am habitually putting to death the deeds prompted by the body, I will live forever.—Romans 8:12–13

I am a debtor, but not to the flesh. I am not obligated to my old carnal nature—to live a life ruled by the standards set up by the dictates of the flesh—because if I live by the dictates of the flesh, I will surely die. But if by the power of the Holy Spirit I am habitually putting to death the deeds prompted by the body, I will live forever.—Romans 8:12–13

I consider that the sufferings of this present time are not worth being compared with the glory that is to be revealed to me and in me and for me and conferred on me.—Romans 8:18

Who (or what) shall ever separate me from Christ's love? Shall suffering and affliction and tribulation? Or calamity and distress? Or persecution or hunger or destitution or peril or sword? It is for His sake I am put to death all day long. Yet amid all these things I am more than a conqueror and gain a surpassing victory through Him who loved me.—Romans 8:35–37

I believe in you, Jesus. I trust you. I rely on you. I will not be put to shame or be disappointed in my expectations.—Romans 9:33

I am now experiencing steadfast patience and endurance and I am able to perform and fully accomplish the will of God. And I receive and carry away and enjoy to the full what is promised.—Hebrews 10:36

My way is not of those who draw back to eternal misery and are destroyed. But I am one of those who believe. I cleave to, trust in, and rely on God, through faith in Jesus Christ. By faith my soul is preserved.—Hebrews 10:39

I choose at all times and for everything to give thanks in the name of my Lord, Jesus Christ, to God the Father.—Ephesians 5:20

I put on God's whole armor. I have an armor of a heavily armed soldier, and God issues it to me. I am able to successfully stand against all the strategies and the deceits of the devil.—Ephesians 6:11

I choose to behave in faith by the practice of patient endurance and waiting, and I am now inheriting the promises.—Hebrews 6:12

Since I have put on God's complete armor, I am able to resist and stand my ground on the evil day of danger. And having done all the crisis demands, I stand firmly in my place.—Ephesians 6:13

It is impossible for God to ever prove false or deceive

me. I have fled to Him for refuge and have received mighty indwelling strength and strong encouragement to grasp and hold fast the hope appointed for me and set before me.—Hebrews 6:18

I have hope as a sure and steadfast anchor of my soul. It cannot slip or break down under me as I step out on it.—Hebrews 6:19

I now seize and hold fast and retain without wavering the hope I cherish and confess. I acknowledge my goal weight of ____pounds, for God who promised it is reliable, sure, and faithful to His Word.—Hebrews 10:23

Books by Marie Chapian:

City Psalms (Moody Press, 1972)
Mind Things (Creation House, 1973)

To My Friend Books, series of 12 Christian gift books
(Successful Living, 1974)

Mustard Seed Library (Creation House, 1974)
The Holy Spirit and Me
I Learn About the Fruit of the Holy Spirit
I learn About the Gifts of the Holy Spirit

*Help Me Remember, Help Me Forget (The Emancipation
    of Robert Sadler)* (Bethany House, 1975)
Of Whom the World Was Not Worthy (Bethany House, 1978)
In the Morning of My Life, the story of Tom Netherton
    (Tyndale House, 1979)
Escape from Rage, the life story of Roger Vann (Bridge
    Publishing, 1981)
Free To Be Thin (Bethany House, 1979)
Telling Yourself the Truth with Dr. William Backus
    (Bethany House, 1980)
Love and Be Loved (Fleming H. Revell, 1983)
Fun To Be Fit (Fleming H. Revell, 1983)
Staying Happy in an Unhappy World (Fleming H. Revell,
    1984)
Why Do I Do What I Don't Want to Do? with Dr. William
    Backus (Bethany House, 1984)
Fun To Be Fit, Blessercize Program available on cassette
    tape and video tape.

Order Marie's books from:

Marie Chapian
P.O. Box 16655
San Diego, CA 92116.

Books by Neva Coyle:

Free To Be Thin, with Marie Chapian, a successful weight-loss plan which links learning how to eat with how to live

Living Free, her personal testimony

Daily Thoughts on Living Free, a devotional

Scriptures for Living Free, a counter-top display book of Scriptures to accompany the devotional

Free To Be Thin Cookbook, a collection of tasty, nutritious recipes complete with the calorie content of each

Free To Be Thin Leader's Kit, a step-by-step guide for organizing and leading an Overeaters Victorious group, including five cassette tapes of instruction

Free To Be Thin Daily Planner, a three-month planner for recording daily thoughts, activities and calorie intake

Tape Albums and Study Guides by Neva Coyle:

The study guides come with the tape albums but may also be ordered separately.

A Seminar on Living Free, a recording of her seminar in which she shares the principles that have helped her break free from a life of misery and self-satisfaction (four cassettes)
Living Free Study Guide, to accompany the tape album

Free To Be Thin (seven cassettes)—Victory, Weight Loss, Deliverance
Free To Be Thin Study Guide No. 1, Getting Started, to be used with the book by the same title, and/or the tape album

Discipline (four cassettes)—A Program for Spiritual Fitness

Free To Be Thin Study Guide No. 2, Discipline, to be used with the book by the same title, and/or the tape album

Abiding (four cassettes)—Honesty in Relationships
Abiding Study Guide

Freedom (four cassettes)—Escape from the Ordinary
Freedom Study Guide

Diligence (four cassettes)—Overcoming Discouragement
Diligence Study Guide

Obedience (four cassettes)—Developing a Listening Heart
Obedience Study Guide

Free To Be Thin Aerobics, available in LP record album with booklet or cassette tape album with booklet.

Detach here

. . . .

For information regarding OVEREATERS VICTORIOUS and for current price lists on other materials, send a business-size, stamped, self-addressed envelope to Overeaters Victorious, Inc., P.O. Box 179, Redlands, CA 92373.

If you would like to receive special mailings concerning Overeaters Victorious seminars in your area, fill out the form below. (*Allow four weeks.*)

Name _____

Address _____

City/State _____ Zip _____

Please print or type.